When East Meets West

An Integrative Guide to Self-Care

Deborah Dolan Hunt, PhD, RN

Rise
An Imprint of Clear Fork Publishing

When East Meets West: An Integrative Guide to Self-Care

Always check with your healthcare provider to discuss safety and possible interactions or precautions!

An Imprint of Clear Fork Publishing

Clear Fork Press
Abilene, Texas
(325) 238-6205
www.clearforkpress.com

Printed and Bound in the United States of America.

ISBN: 979-8-3496-2112-3

To my darling granddaughters, Kaylie Ryan and Alexis Grace. You are a blessing and a joy and I love you more and more every day. To my mom and beloved father for supporting me in following my dreams, and to my children who generously contributed to this book. They are my "true north" and are always there to support and encourage me.

To my friends and family old and new, near and far who have shared my journey.

And to all the readers of this book I hope it will inspire you to develop your individual health and wellness plan in consultation with your healthcare provider.

To Callie ---my friend and publisher who has the kindest heart and has spent countless hours collaborating on this special book.

Introduction

There are many potential health benefits of essential oils, herbal teas, and self-care practices. This book will provide information about various essential oils, herbal teas, tinctures, superfoods, and other self-care practices along with recommendations for use and precautions to follow. It is important to note that this book is informational, and one should consult with their healthcare provider to explore the benefits and risks before incorporating any of these self-care measures. These practices are not meant to replace conventional medical practices which are considered Western practices, but to complement care. Although some individuals choose solely alternative practices, many choose an integrative approach that incorporates conventional (Western) with complementary practices (Eastern). Somewhat akin to East meets West.

When I was in grad school, I took a course in Complementary Medicine and it literally changed the way I viewed health and wellness. During that semester I learned about meditation, journaling, therapeutic touch, essential oils, chakras, and healing with crystals and I incorporated these into my daily life. Learning how to meditate helped me to deal with stress which sometimes resulted in a panic attack. At the time I didn't realize I was having panic attacks when my heart would beat rapidly and I would feel a sense of impending doom. Although I was quite young but because I was a critical care nurse, I thought I had a serious cardiac issue. After a visit to the cardiologist and a series of tests, I was relieved to be told that everything was normal. At some point I realized it was anxiety and once I knew the signs, I would meditate and do some breathing exercises and I was able to prevent the panic attack. This was very empowering and enlightening. The practice of therapeutic touch and the use of energy fields intrigued me so I continued to do research on it and incorporated it into my health and wellness regime. I used it on my family and my kids would ask me to do my "magic" on them when they were not feeling well. Therapeutic Touch is similar to Reiki but you do not actually touch the person but use your hands to unruffle energy blockages and restore balance. Recently, I did therapeutic touch on my friend's dog who had lost his hearing and the next day Nitro could hear some noises. Everyone was surprised, including me. I always enjoyed drinking tea and some herbal teas but never really thought about the health benefits until my daughter started sharing information about the myriad benefits of herbal teas. I started researching and learning more about teas and eventually created my own blend of moonshine tea that I consume on a daily basis. When I was in my doctoral program, I took a class on hypnosis and learned about the therapeutic effects of this practice and incorporated self-hypnosis into my life. I used essential oils sporadically and as they gained in popularity, I started researching the various essential oils and created my own special blend for my personal use. I firmly believe that each individual person should develop their own individualized and integrative approach to health and wellness. These practices can truly make a difference. You might not prevent certain diseases but you can certainly manage them better with a holistic approach.

Take, for example, Hypertension (high blood pressure) depending on your blood pressure you may need to take medication as there are serious complications to uncontrolled hypertension. However, if you take a holistic approach with healthy eating, exercise, meditation, essential oils such as lavender, and green tea you will be better able to control your high blood pressure, and potentially require less medication while preventing serious complications.

This introductory book contains information about a majority of complementary or alternative medicine and folk healing that can be incorporated in your daily health and wellness regime. I strongly recommend you consult with your healthcare provider and do your own research before you incorporate them.

Maslow's Hierarchy of Needs

Nourishing one's body, mind, and spirit is vital for well-being. Incorporating some or all the practices in this book may help you reach the goals listed in Maslow's Hierarchy of Needs that can guide one in the health and wellness journey. The hierarchy is depicted as a triangle that has five levels built upon one another. They include physiological, psychological, and self-fulfillment needs. The most basic needs listed as the bottom include food, water, warmth, and rest. The second level is security and safety. The third level is intimate relations and friends. The fourth level is esteem and accomplishments, and the fifth and top level is self-fulfillment when you reach your full potential.

Nourishing One's Body

Herbal Teas

By Meaghan Hunt

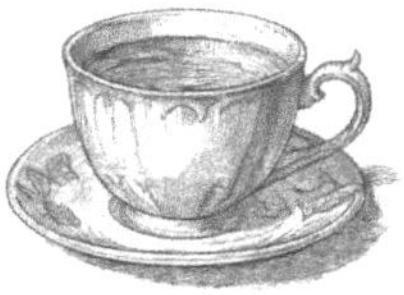

A popular method of extracting the medicinal properties and flavors of herbs for consuming is by the process of infusion. An infusion is made by steeping plant material in water for a certain length of time. For tougher parts of herbs (roots, seeds, etc.), a decoction may be made of the herb by simmering in water over a longer period. Most of the herbs mentioned in this section are leaves or flowers and will work just fine as an infusion. Many people choose to strain their teas before drinking but, in most cases, this is optional.

Infusion (Steeping)

- Add 1 tsp to 1 tbsp of dried herb for each cup of water. A glass mason jar with a sealable lid is best, as it will seal in the plant's volatile oils and ensure medicinal properties are kept intact. A French press or simply a mug with a plate or flat object over it works fine too!
- Pour boiling or hot water over herbs
- Cover your tea and let steep for 5 to 30 minutes
- Strain, sweeten with honey or sugar, or drink as is!

Decoction (Simmering)

- Add 1 tsp to 1 tbsp of dried herb for each cup of water. A pot with a tight-fitting lid is ideal.
- Simmer herbs and water together, covered, for around 20 to 30 minutes.

- Strain, add sweetener of choice, or drink as is!

These methods are a great way to begin experiencing herbal teas but feel free to experiment as you'd like; stronger teas can be made using more plant material per cup of water or by letting them steep longer, or weaker by using less material and shorter steep time. The more you experiment, the better sense you will gain of the herbs and methods best fit for you and your loved ones!

There are many brands of packaged teas that can be purchased, for example:

- Yogi
- Twinings
- Celestial Seasons

Loose teas can be purchased from the following shops (this is just a sample):

- Mountain Rose Herbs
- Adagio Teas

- The Tea Spot
- Matcha Source
- Verdant Tea

Caffeine has been touted to have both positive and negative effects but is considered safe with moderate consumption. Moderate consumption of up to 400mg of caffeine is safe. However, in some health conditions caffeine should be avoided so it is best to check with your healthcare provider.

Herbal teas have many benefits but further research is necessary to support these benefits. The following section contains a brief overview of a variety of teas and what ailments they may be beneficial in treating.

Lemon Balm (Melissa officinalis)

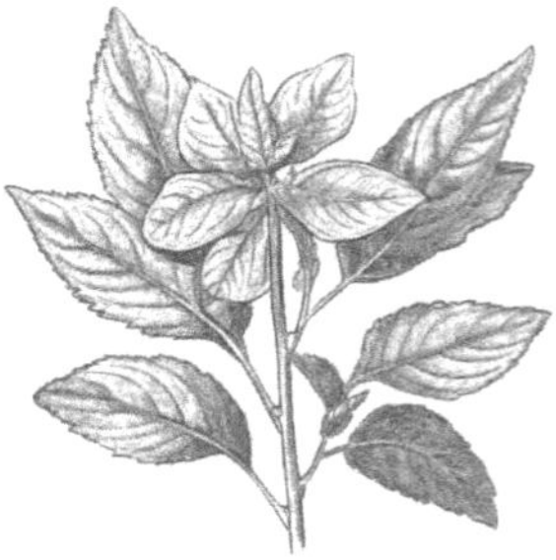

Caffeine free

- Lemon balm is a mint family herb known for its calmative properties

- It is antispasmodic, relaxing both the stomach and the nervous system
- It is antiviral and often used in the treatment of herpes, colds, and flu
- The herb can be used as a mild sedative for insomnia
- Can be drunk throughout the day as a tonic for stress and anxiety

Red Raspberry Leaf (Rubus idaeus)

Caffeine free

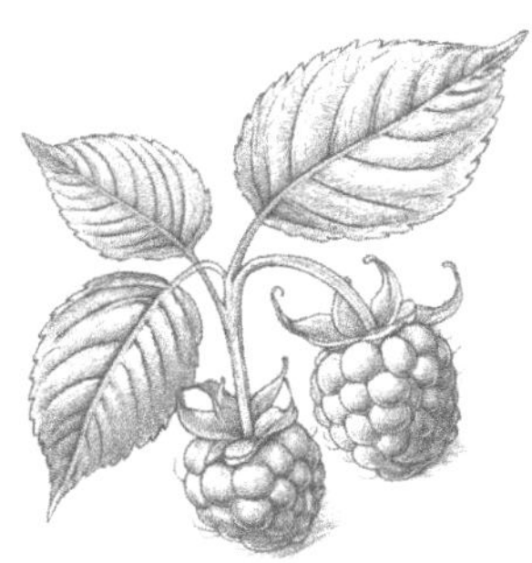

- Red raspberry leaf is an herb known for its role in aiding the reproductive and genitourinary systems
- This herb is an abundant source of iron, niacin, and manganese
- Due to the astringent properties, this herb can be helpful for inflamed

mouth and gums Red Raspberry Leaf (Rubus idaeus)

- Due to its high mineral content, the tea can be drunk as a tonic to support bleeding during menstruation

Chamomile (Matricaria recutita)

Caffeine free

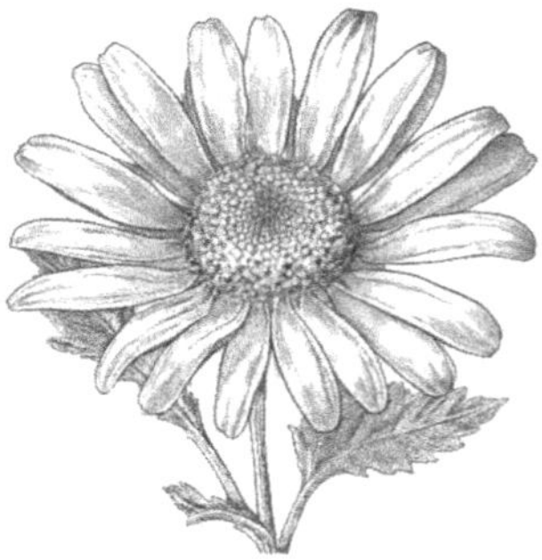

- Chamomile is a highly accessible herb noted for its gentle, calmative effects
- This herb, due to its bitter properties, is a wonderful digestive aid Diaphoretic, thus induces sweating when treating fevers
- Chamomile can also be used in cases of mild insomnia for its positive effects on the nervous system

Spearmint (Mentha spicata)

Caffeine free

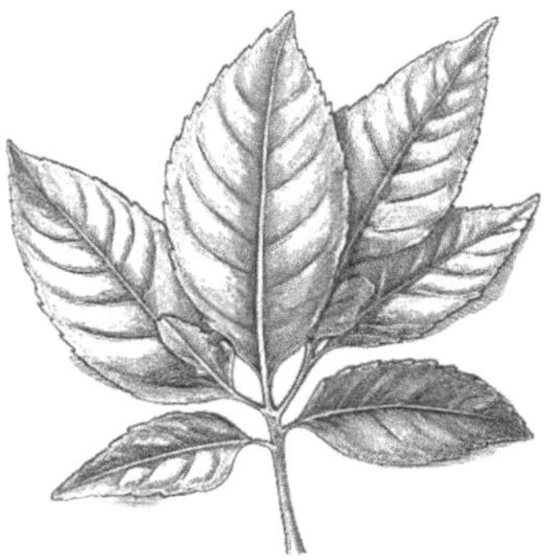

- Spearmint is a mint family herb that aids in digestion, focus, & cooling down
- Can be used to freshen breath
- Especially useful for cases of nausea or motion sickness
- Aids in alleviation of bloating and gas
- Can be used for sweating out fever or colds

Lavender (Lavandula spp.)

Caffeine free

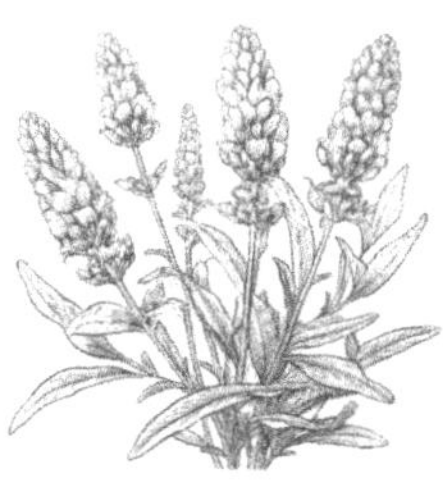

- Lavender is an herb widely known for its relaxing effects on the nervous system
- Works well in cases of mild depression

- Aids in alleviating tension, sleeping problems, and stress
- A little goes a long way, this is a wonderful herb to add to a tea blend in small doses

Corn Silk (Zea mays)

Caffeine free

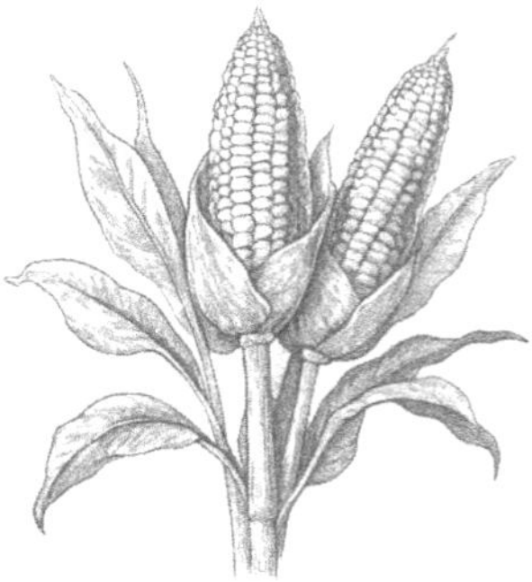

- Corn silk is a highly accessible medicine that you can gather it simply from the remnants of your dinner
- Makes a fantastic tonic for urinary tract because of demulcent and diuretic effects
- Soothes inflammation in the urinary system. Can aid in cases of bed-wetting

Holy Basil (Ocimum sanctum)

Caffeine free

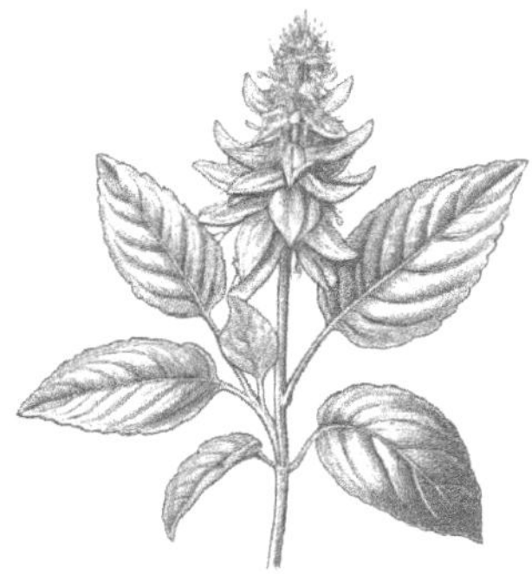

- Holy Basil, otherwise known as Tulsi, is a plant revered for its many medicinal properties
- Helps to reduce inflammation thus aiding in alleviation of pain
- Helps to strengthen the digestive system Stimulates immunity thus helping to ward off colds and flu
- Adaptogenic properties make this plant a wonderful daily tonic

Nettle (Urtica dioica)

Caffeine free

- This herb is commonly known as stinging nettle due to its effect on the skin when coming in contact

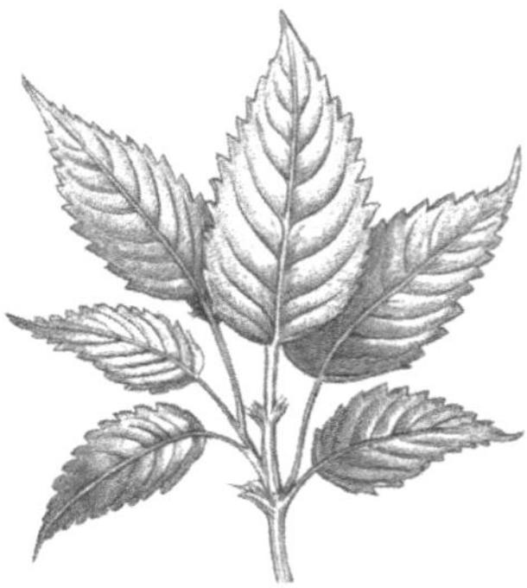

- When brewed into a tea however, it is high in vitamins and minerals such as calcium, magnesium, iron, potassium, silicon, & zinc Used to support circulation
- Supports adrenal and kidney function
- Useful in treatment of arthritis
- Used in treatment of allergies

Oats (Avena sativa)

Caffeine free

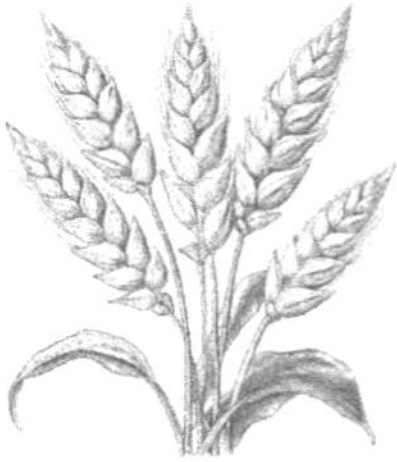

- The milky tops of oats make for the most nourishing of teas, though the stalks or grass are useful as well
- Oats make for a great daily tonic, especially in cases of extreme stress or anxiety
- Can enhance sexual energy and libido

- Brew a cup of this (or combine with lemon balm & chamomile) to quell an irritated or off mood

Cinnamon (Cinnamomum verum)

Caffeine free

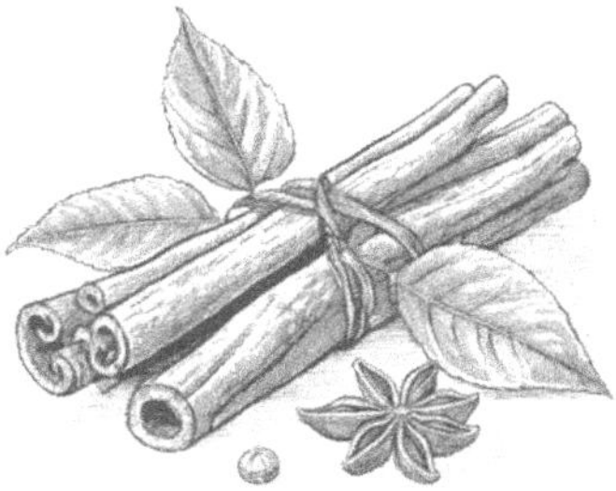

- May lower cholesterol
- Antioxidant
- Lower blood sugar
- You can make cinnamon tea with cinnamon sticks and boiling water. Let steep for 10 minutes.

Blueberry (Vaccinium corymbosum)

Caffeine free

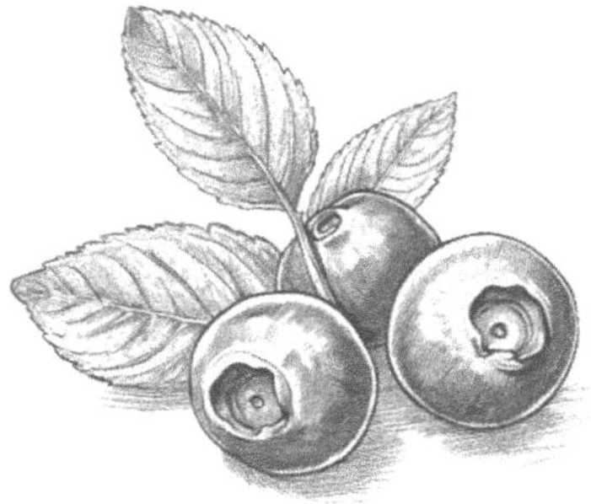

- Rich in antioxidants
- Improved Heart Health

- Improved Brain Function
- Strengthen Immune System
- May decrease risk of Type 2 Diabetes
- Steep blueberry leaves in 8 oz's of hot water for 30 minutes

Kombucha Tea

Caffeine

Kombucha tea dates to ancient Northeast China (200 B.C.) and was believed to have healing properties.

- Supports gut health and digestion
- Immune support
- Promote well-being
- Improve vitality

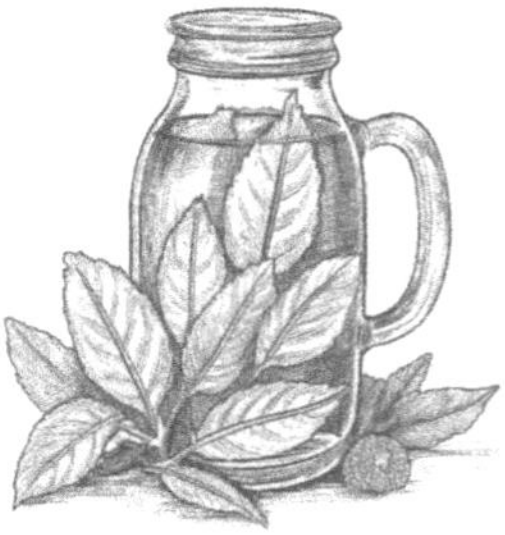

Kombucha tea is a fermented drink which can be made with green or black tea, sugar, bacteria, and yeast. Because it is fermented, you must be careful and be sure to follow a trusted recipe.

Dandelion (pu gong ying) Root Tea (Taraxacum officinale)

Caffeine free

- May have diuretic properties
- Dried leaves may be used for skin ailments
- Aids in digestion
- Anti-diabetic properties
- Liver health
- May have anti-cancer properties
- Weight loss
- UTI prevention

Flowers and Leaves: Wash, then let steep in hot water for 15-20 minutes.

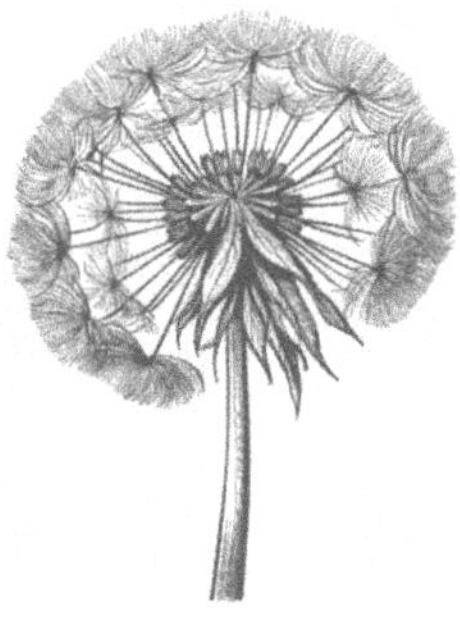

Roots: Wash thoroughly, chop into fine pieces, and heat on high in an oven for about two hours. Steep 1-2 teaspoons in hot water for about 10 minutes.

Precautions: *May interact with certain medications.*

. . .

Rooibos (Aspalathus linearis)

Caffeine free

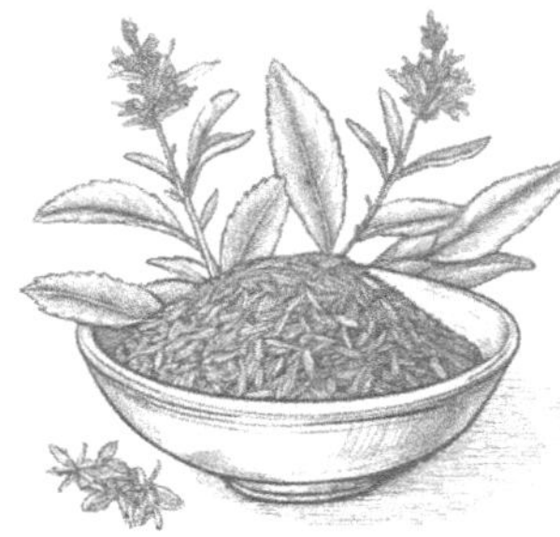

- Antioxidant
- Heart Health
- Diabetes Management
- Weight loss
- Wrinkle reduction

Leaves are fermented and steeped in hot water.

Green Tea (Camellia sinensis)

Caffeine free

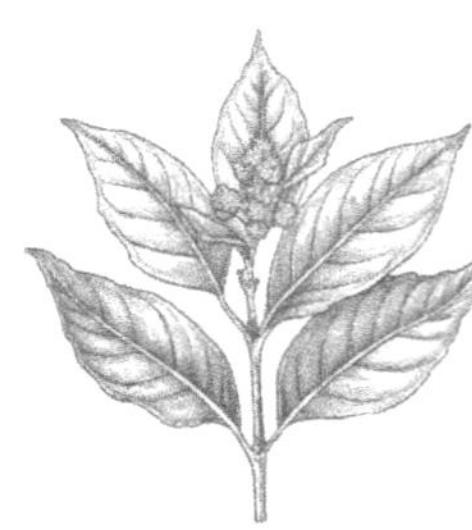

- Heart disease
- Cancer
- Genital warts
- Ovarian and Uterine Cancer

Leaves are fermented and steeped in hot water. Drink in moderation

Rose Hip (Rosa canina)

Caffeine free

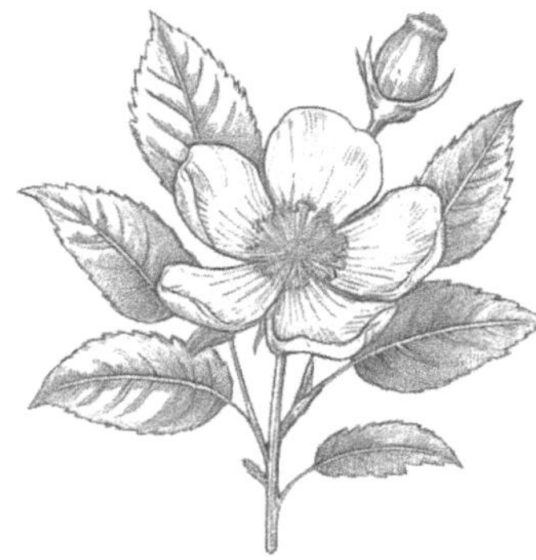

- May support immune system
- Heart Health
- Weight loss
- Help to manage Type 2 Diabetes
- May improve skin and prevent wrinkles

Rose Hip tea can be made with the fruit of the rose petal or with dried rose hips. Tea should steep in hot water for 10-15 minutes.

Precautions: May cause nausea/vomiting. Do not use it in Pregnancy or when breastfeeding.

Peppermint Tea (Mentha piperita L.)

Caffeine free

- Antibacterial properties
- Treats nausea and abdominal pain
- Mental clarity

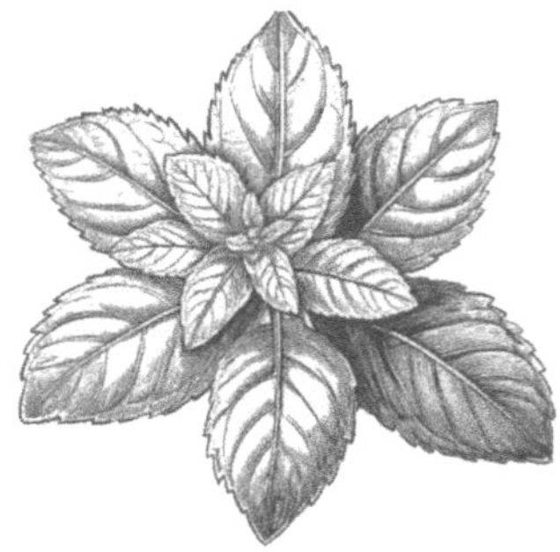

- Antioxidant
- Headaches
- Nasal congestion

May use fresh or dried peppermint. Steep in hot water for 5 minutes

Ginger (Zingiberaceae)

Caffeine free

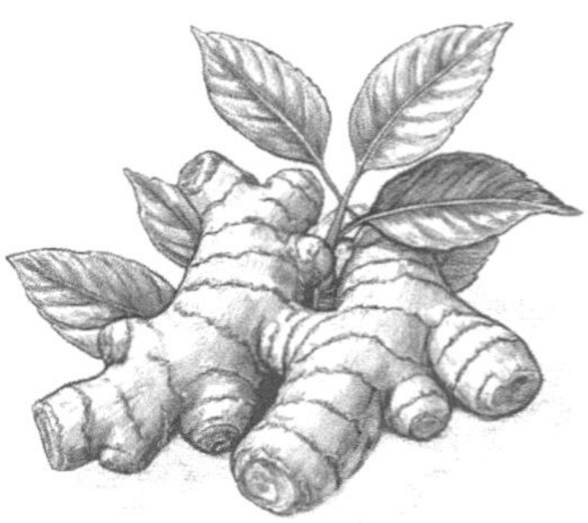

- Nausea
- Motion sickness
- Heart health
- Weight control
- Blood pressure
- Blood sugar
- Pain Relief
- Immune support

Use fresh ginger that is cleaned, peeled, and sliced. Boil for 20 minutes. Add lemon or honey.

. . .

Hibiscus (Hibiscus Sabdariffa)

Caffeine free

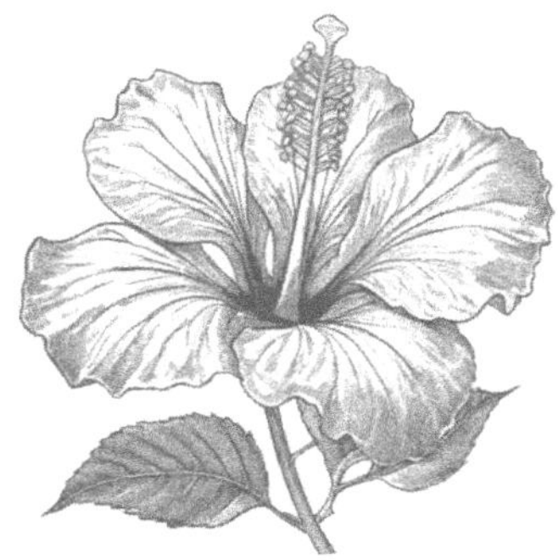

Hibiscus tea can be made by steeping 1.5 teaspoons of dried hibiscus in 1 cup of boiling water for five to 10 minutes.

- High blood pressure
- Weight loss
- Diabetes management
- May help to lower cholesterol

Precautions: May interfere with other medications (hypertensives, antidiabetics, and birth control). Limit to 2-3 cups per day.

Echinacea Tea (Purple Coneflower) (Echinacea purpurea)

Caffeine free

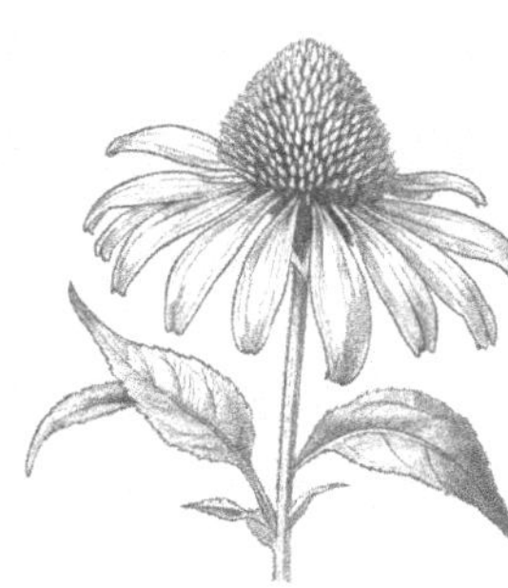

Steep upper plants or roots in boiling water and let steep for 5-10 minutes.

- Antioxidant
- Lowers blood sugar
- Skin conditions

- Anxiety
- Boosts immune system

Precautions:

May cause nausea, dizziness, rashes, and hives

Chai Tea

Caffeine but may find decaffeinated brands

- Blood pressure
- Blood sugar
- Energy
- Antioxidants
- Heart Health
- Weight loss
- Brain health

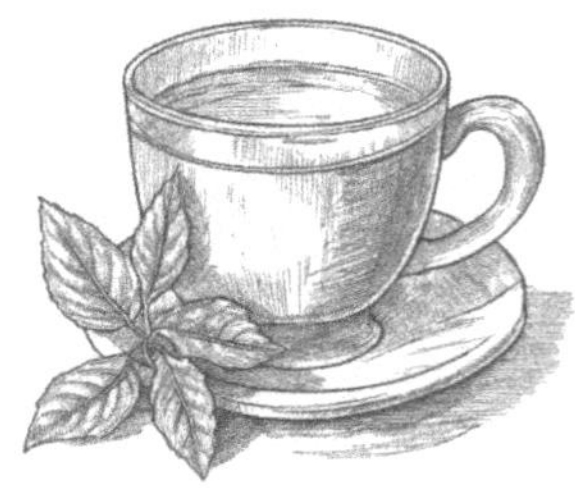

Precautions: Chai tea has caffeine and is often made with milk and sugar but can be made with skim, almond milk, and raw honey.

Licorice Root Tea (Glycyrrhiza glabra)

Caffeine free

Steep licorice root in hot water for 30 minutes

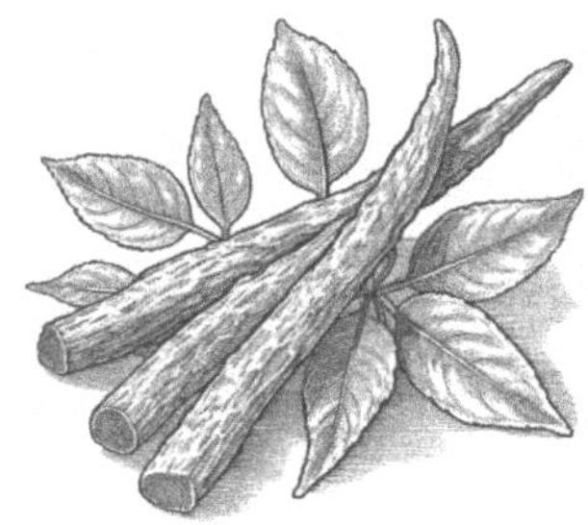

- •Skin conditions
- •Acid Reflux
- •Peptic Ulcer
- •Anticancer
- •Upper respiratory
- •Cavities

Precautions: Licorice Root tea has many benefits but should also be used with caution.

May have serious interactions with blood pressure medications, blood thinners. cholesterol lowering medications, including statins, diuretics, estrogen-based contraceptives, and nonsteroidal anti-inflammatory drugs (NSAIDs).

My Tea Blend (Deb's Moonshine Tea)

You can experiment with your teas and blend them. Just be sure to do some research on the benefits, uses, and precautions. Every morning I make a

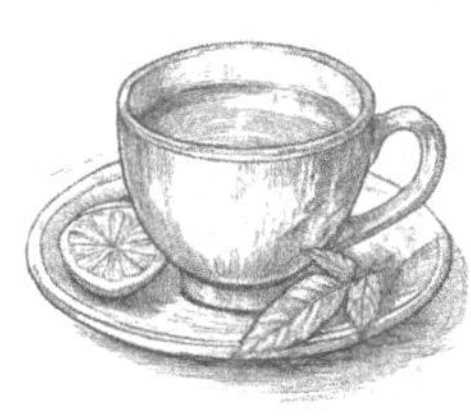

mason jar of blended teas (3-4 different ones) and add raw honey, a few drops of elderberry, sprinkled with ground turmeric, cinnamon, and cardamom.

My blends include:

- Green tea Kombucha
- Blueberry tea
- Lemon Ginger
- Dandelion Root
- Chai tea
- Chamomile
- Peppermint

Bibliography[1]

Essential Oils

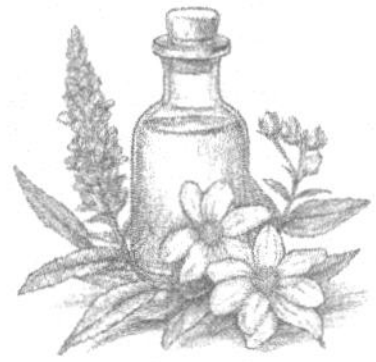

Essential oils are derived from various plants made through a process of distillation with water or steam. Essential oils are used in Aromatherapy, and some may be applied topically but need to be diluted in distilled water or a carrier oil such as jojoba. There are various ways to use it as aromatherapy. You may purchase a diffuser or place several drops on a piece of cotton.

Precautions

- Do not use if allergic to the essential

oil of choice or plants that the oil is derived from

- Do a small skin test prior to use
- Avoid excessive use
- Discontinue if sensitivity occurs
- Do not use if pregnant or breastfeeding until consulting with healthcare provider
- Do not use on children until consulting with healthcare provider
- May be harmful to pets. Consult with your vet.
- Essential oils should not be ingested unless directed by your healthcare provider.
- Do not place in ears or eyes
- It's also important to purchase oils from a reputable shop
- Use only as directed
- Check with your healthcare provider about any potential interactions due to current prescribed medications and health status.
- Use a reputable source to purchase quality essential oils.

Although there are approximately 100 essential oils (see reference page)* we will focus on the most used ones.

Many essential oils can be blended; however, it is important to read up on the various oils and how to blend them.

Body Sprays

- Fill a 4-ounce spray bottle with distilled water (3.5 Oz)
- Add 15-30 drops of your selected essential oil (be sure to check any precautions)

Baths

- Essential oils should be placed in a "carrier oil" such as jojoba or olive oil prior to placing in a bath
- May add 5-10 drops to a tablespoon of oil and then add to bath

---

* *See reference list for additional guidelines

- Suggested oils - lavender, ylang ylang, geranium, and grapefruit

Aromatherapy

- If using a diffuser follow directions for the specific diffuser
- May also be placed in boiling water by adding several drops of your favorite essential oil.

Lavender Oil:

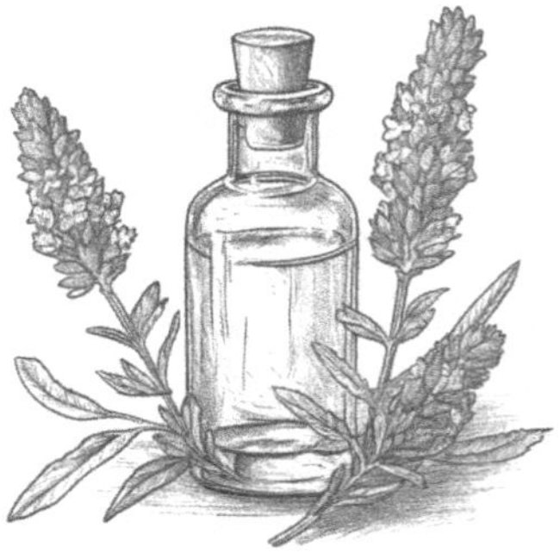

- Lavender is an essential oil used for relaxation and stress reduction
- It can also treat headaches and pain
- It can be added to a diffuser, or a few drops can be placed on pillows
- It can also be added to distilled water

and used as a body spray or room freshener

- A few drops can also be added to hand lotion

Rose Oil:

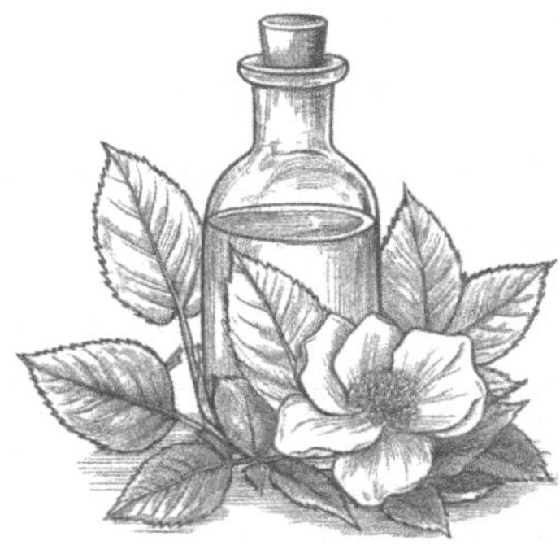

- Rose is an essential oil that may used to treat depression
- Can be used for pain
- Can be used in baths
- For lung ailments ~place 3-5 drops in a bowl of near boiling water and breathe in the vapors
- For skin ailments~ 1-2 drops may be applied to affected area

Precautions: Check with healthcare provider for use during pregnancy

Lemon Oil

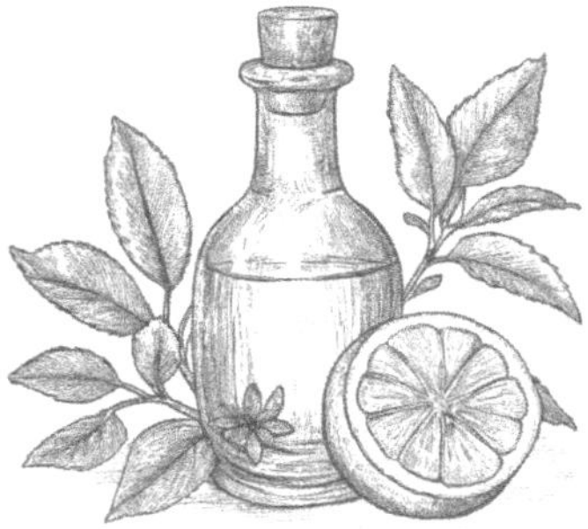

- Aromatherapy
- Skin Care
- Hair Conditioner
- Cleaning products

Precautions: Check with healthcare provider if pregnant, Avoid direct sunlight if using topically

Orange Oil

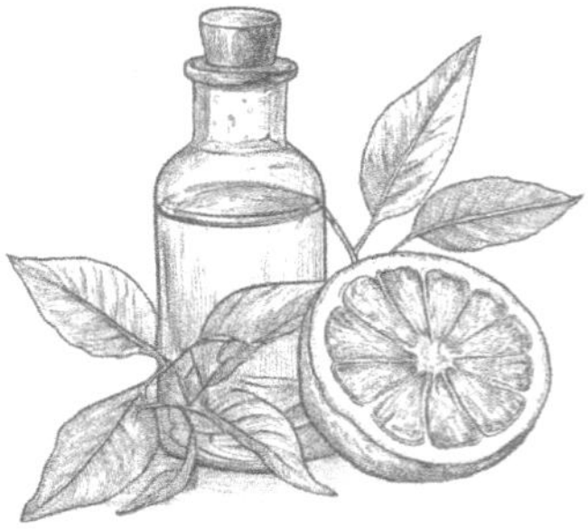

- Reduces inflammation
- Disinfects wounds
- May be used for depression and anxiety
- Treat acne
- Increase libido
- May have a calming effect

Precautions: Photosensitivity

Bergamot Oil:

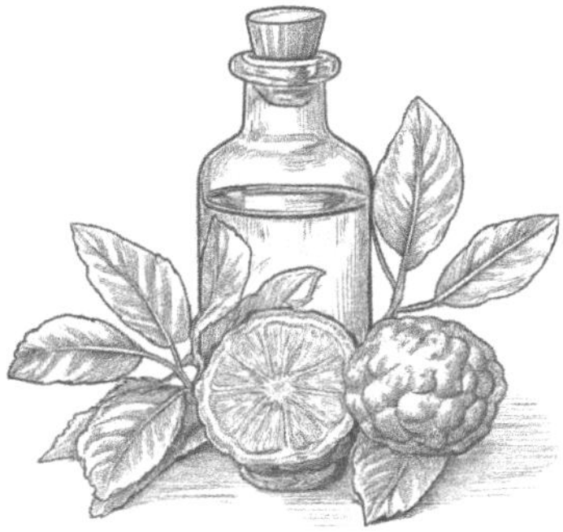

- Reduces pain
- Improves circulation
- Decreases stress and anxiety
- Skin Care and Relaxation
- a vaporizer for chest congestion

Precautions: *Photosensitivity*

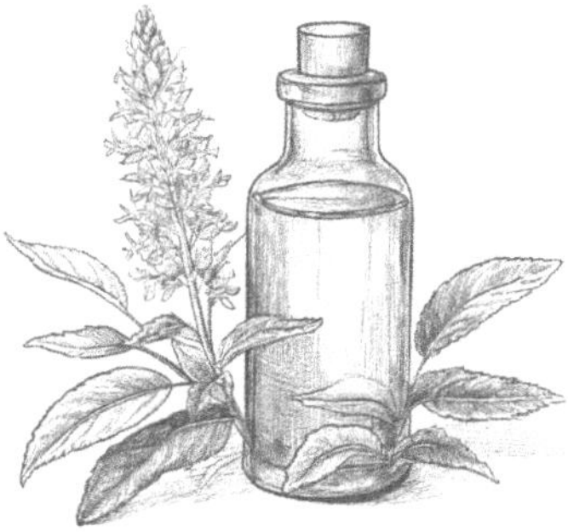

Clary Sage Oil:

- Balance female hormones
- Menstrual cramps
- Menopause
- Aphrodisiac and Improve mood
- Headaches and Depression

Precautions: *Photosensitivity, Do not use during pregnancy or when consuming alcohol*

Frankincense Oil:

- Relieves stress
- Regulates menstruation
- Skin Care
- Relieves stress
- May boost immune system

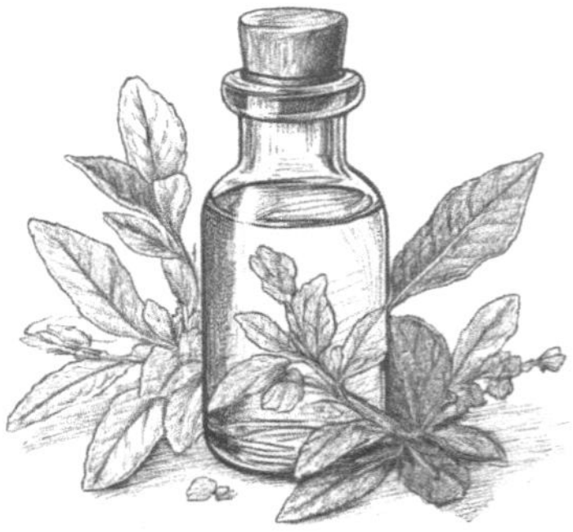

Precautions: *Do not use during pregnancy*

Tea Tree Oil

- Acne
- Dandruff
- Lice
- Nail fungus

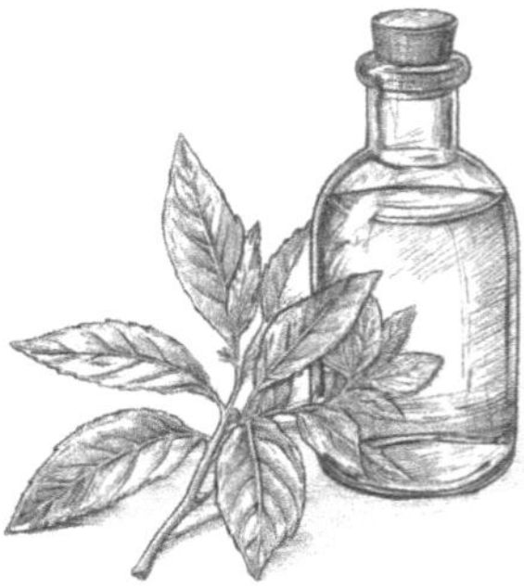

Precautions: *Toxic if ingested*

Roman Chamomile Oil

- Allergies, Arthritis
- Colic and Nausea
- Promotes sleep
- Stress and Strains
- Skin care (cuts, insect bites), PMS

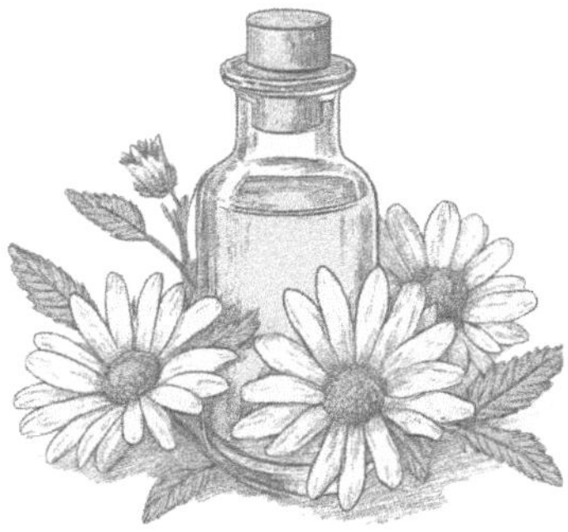

Precautions: *May cause dermatitis*

Cypress Oil

- Wound healing
- Decreases spasms
- Increases urination
- Relieves stress
- Regulates blood flow
- Clears chest congestion

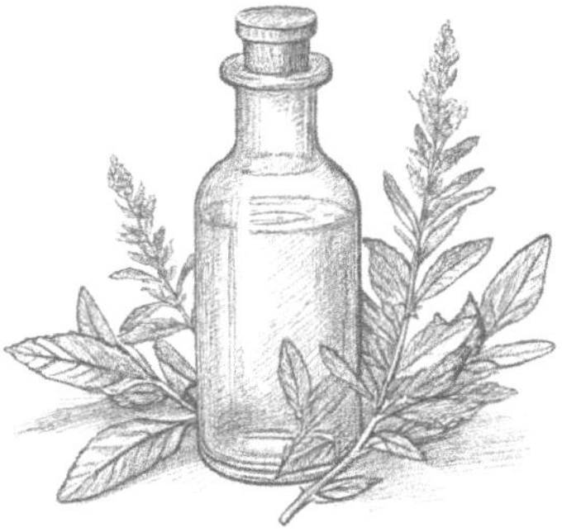

Precautions: *Avoid during pregnancy and breastfeeding*

Ginger Oil:

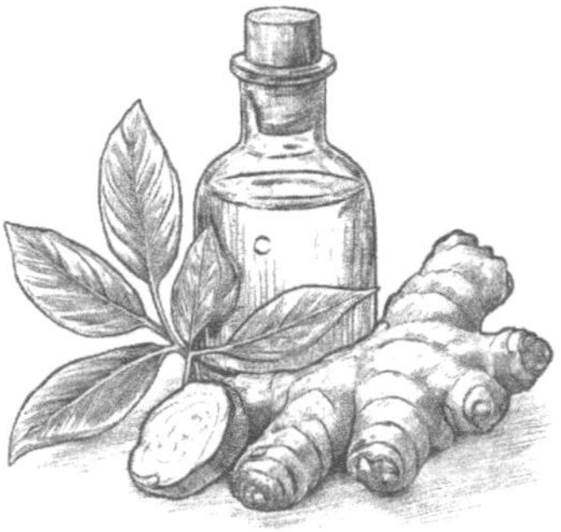

- Digestion
- Infections
- Expectorant (ginger tea)
- Anxiety
- Nausea (ginger tea)
- Aphrodisiac
- Muscle cramps and menstrual pains

Precautions: *Do not take if pregnant, Consult healthcare provider if taking blood thinners*

Ylang-Ylang Oil

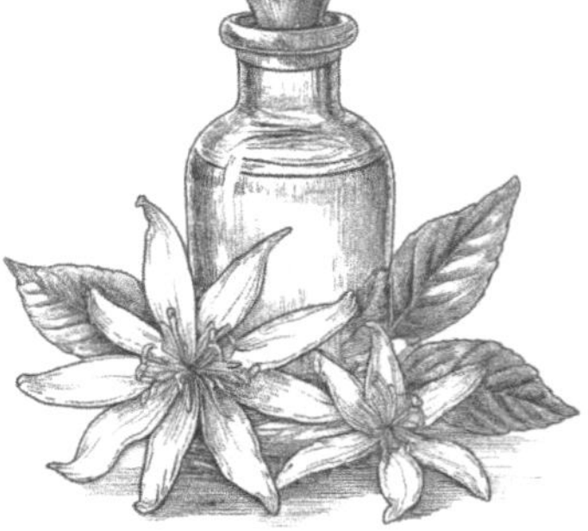

- Calming
- Balances hormones
- Healthy skin and hair

Precautions: *Long term use may result in skin sensitivities*

Eucalyptus Oil:

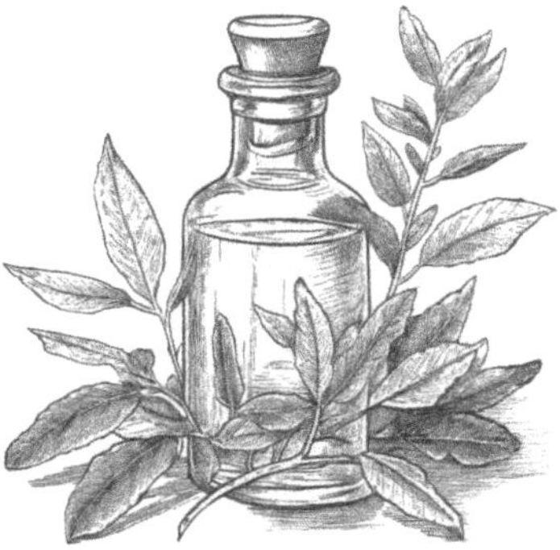

- Wound Healing
- Clear congestion
- Oral care
- Lice
- Pain
- Intestinal health
- Help to regulate blood sugar

Precautions: *May result in toxicity if taking more than recommended amount*

Patchouli Oil:

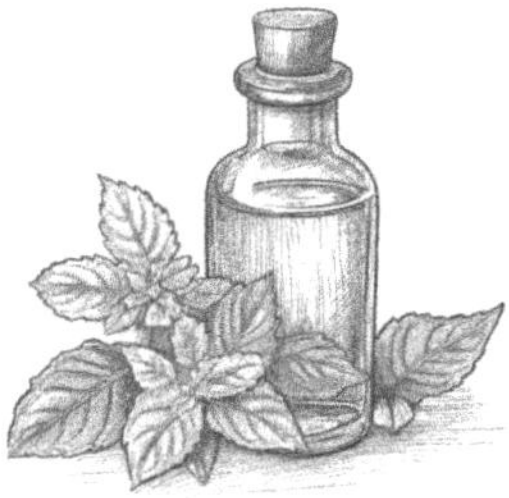

- Infections, Treat fevers
- Astringent, Aphrodisiac
- Stimulates circulation
- Stimulates urination

Precautions: *When used in Aromatherapy may be irritating*

Lemongrass Oil:

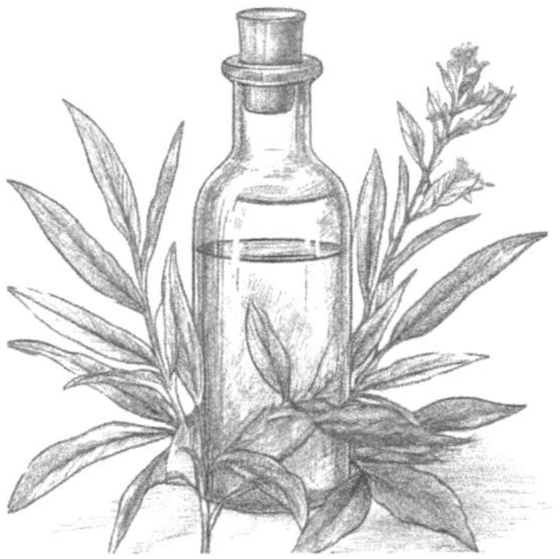

- Digestion
- High blood pressure
- Fever
- Achy joints
- Colds
- Muscle pain

Precautions: *Discontinue use if sensitivity develops*

Peppermint Oil:

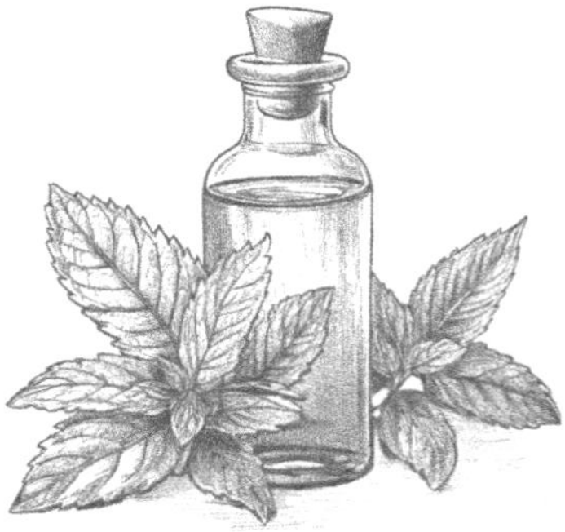

- Digestive aid, UTI
- Oral care
- Stress, Pain
- Skin Care
- Improves circulation
- Immunity booster

Precautions: *May cause heartburn, allergic reactions, and headaches*

Spearmint Oil:

- Antibacterial
- Digestion
- Colds and flu
- Pain relief
- Stress, Depression

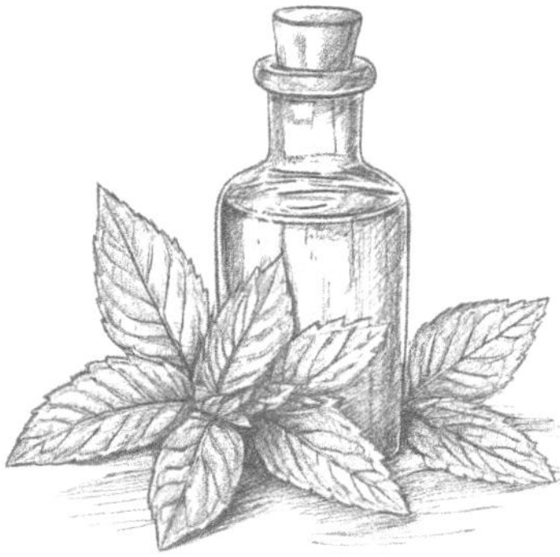

Precautions:

Discontinue if sensitivity develops

Wintergreen Oil:

- Pain
- Spasms
- Arthritis
- Muscle relaxant
- Flatulence
- Increases urination

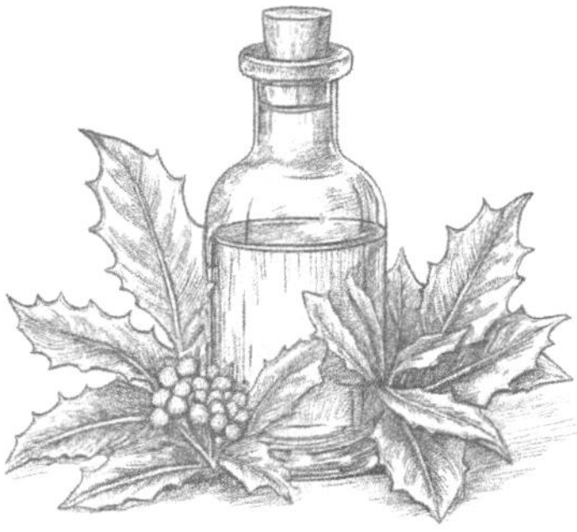

Precautions: *It should never be ingested or used in Aromatherapy*

Vetiver Oil:

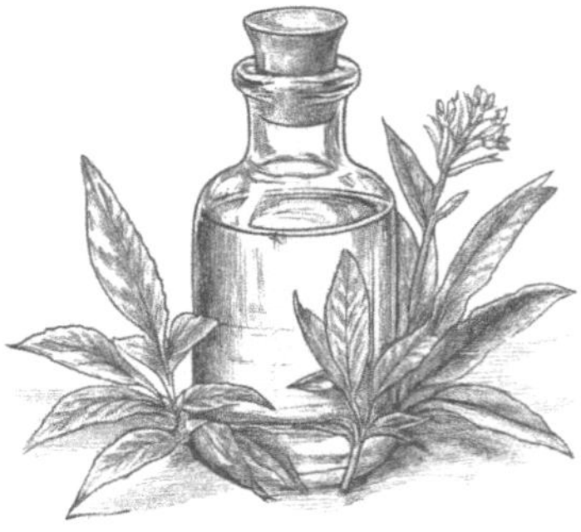

- Inflammation
- Scars
- Aphrodisiac
- Stress
- Insomnia
- Wound healing
- Dry skin

Precautions: *Discontinue use if sensitivity occurs*

Vanilla Oil:

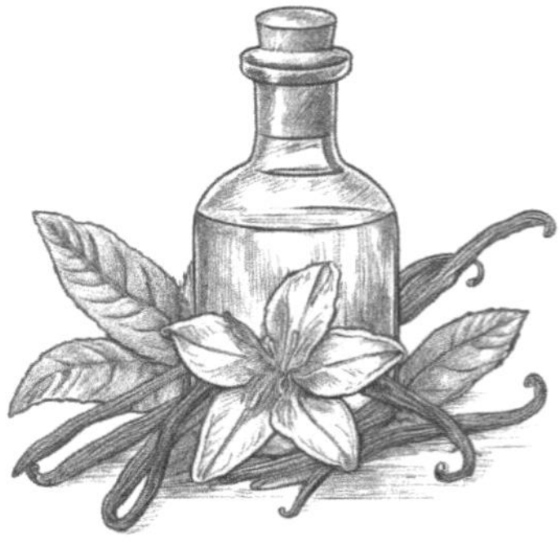

- Antioxidant
- Aphrodisiac
- Fever
- Sedation, Sleep
- Enhances libido
- Depression

Precautions: *Discontinue use if sensitivity occurs*

Geranium Oil
Rose Geranium Oil

Geranium oil is derived from the plant Pelargonium graveolens.

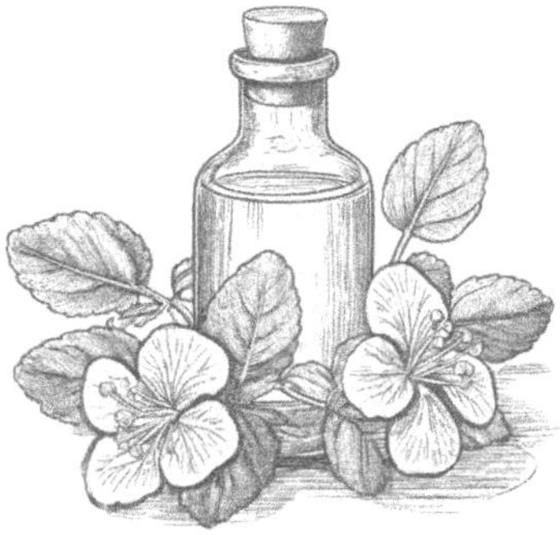

- Acne
- Edema
- Diabetes particularly hyperglycemia
- Nasovastibulitis
- Infections
- Neurodegenerative Disorders
- Stress and anxiety
- Menopause
- Allergies

Precautions: May develop allergic reactions. If pregnant or nursing, check with a healthcare provider.

Grapefruit Oil

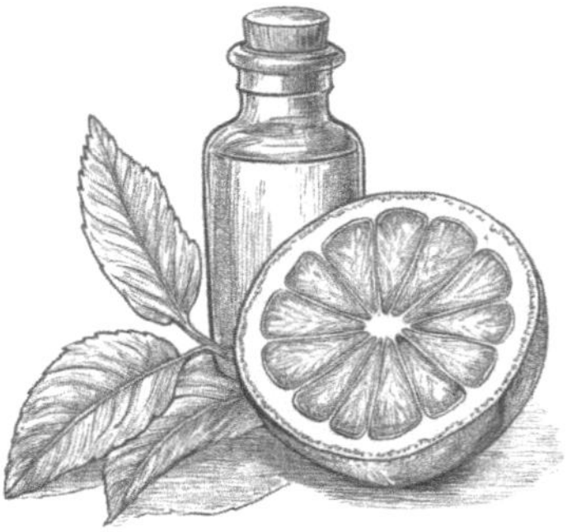

- Appetite suppressant
- Weight loss
- Mood enhancement
- Stress
- Blood pressure
- Antimicrobial
- Acne

Precautions: Do not use it if pregnant or nursing until you consult with your healthcare provider.

Lime Oil

Lime oil is made from the zest of the lime.

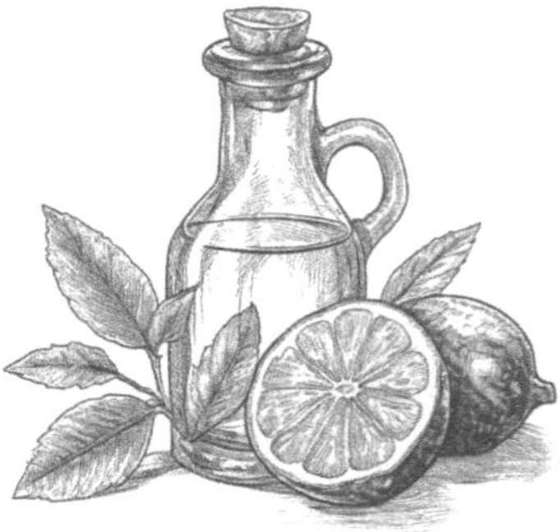

- Antioxidant
- Decreases inflammation
- Weight loss

- Diabetes risk
- Cholesterol
- Mood
- Detoxifier
- Acne
- Pain

Precautions: Although small amounts may be used in cooking, always check with your healthcare provider.

Rosemary Oil (Rosmarinus officinalis)

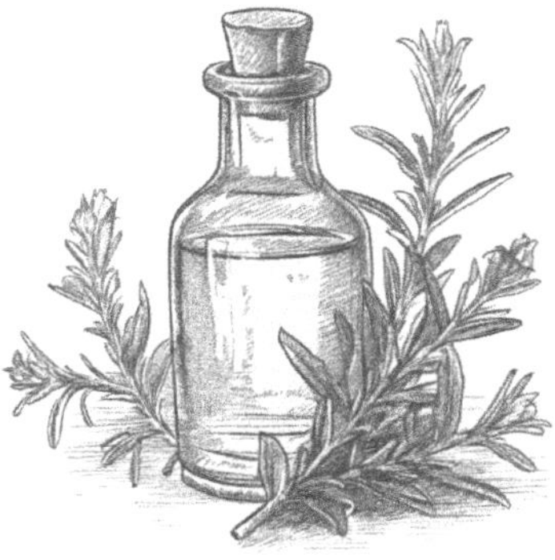

- Brain function
- Hair growth
- Pain relief
- Stress relief
- Bug repellent
- Decreased inflammation

Precautions: Do not use it if you have bleeding disorders or in pregnancy.

White Camphor Oil

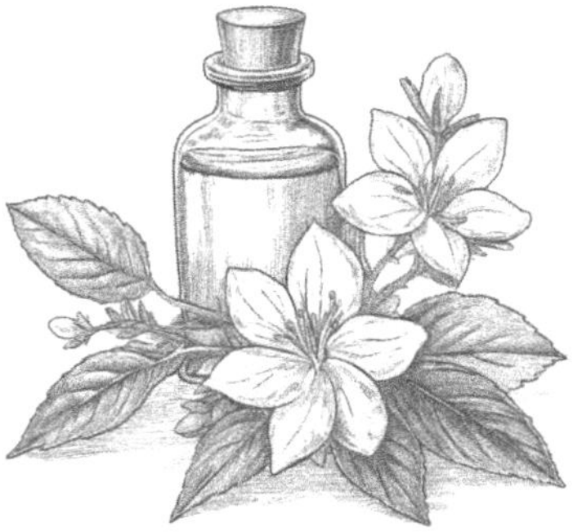

- Pain
- Skin irritations
- Headaches
- Coughs
- Superficial burns
- Chronic Diseases

Precautions: Do not apply to open wounds. Do not ingest.

Fennel Oil

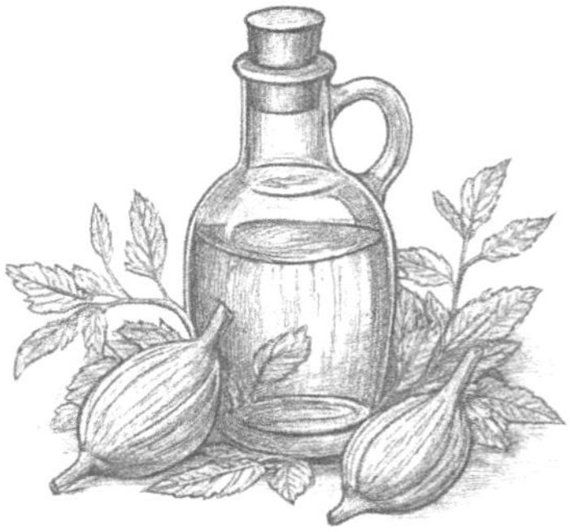

- Wound healing
- Spasms
- Laxative
- Menstruation
- Purifies Blood
- Chronic cough

Precautions: May cause hallucinations. Do not use any history of epilepsy.

Helichrysum (Helichrysum italicum)

Essential oils are made from the leaves and stems of the plant.

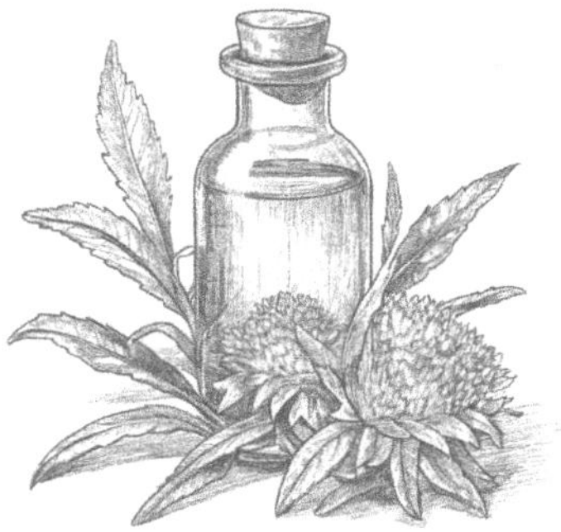

- Allergies
- Prevent infections
- Colds
- Prevent weight gain
- Skin irritations
- Wound healing
- Digestive disorders
- Candida
- Gallbladder disorders
- Inflammation

Precautions: May interfere with liver enzymes. May cause contact dermatitis.

Mandarin Oil

Made from the rind of a mandarin

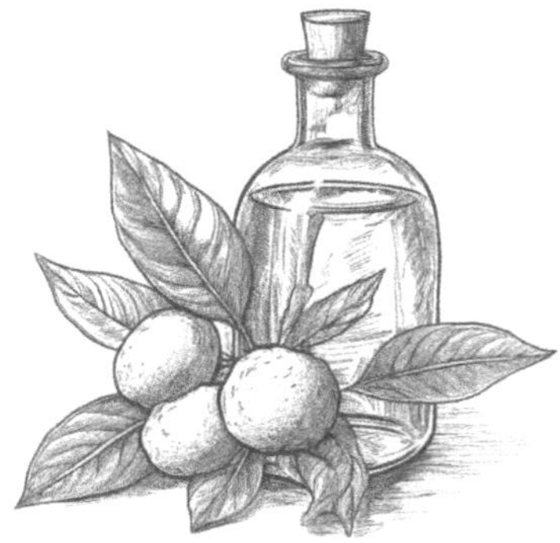

- Prevents infections
- Relieves spasms
- Improves circulation
- Removes toxins
- Aids digestion
- Stomach disorders
- Sedative effect

Precautions: *May cause photosensitivity.*

Neroli (Citrus aurantium var. amara) Orange Blossom

The oil is extracted from the flowers of bitter orange trees.

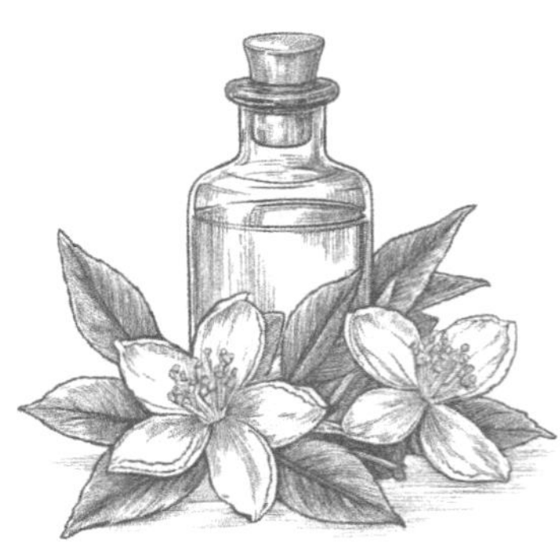

- Stress and anxiety
- Menopause
- Depression
- Seizures

- High blood pressure
- Acne and skin irritations

Precautions: *May cause photosensitivity. Do not use tanning booths.*

End Notes: *

---

* https://naha.org/explore aromatherapy/about-aromatherapy/what-are-essential-oils

https://www.organicfacts.net/health-benefits/essential-oils/health-benefits-of-rose-essential-oil.html

https://www.livestrong.com/article/251041-what-are-the-benefits-of-rose-essential-oil/

http://www.sustainablebabysteps.com/rose-essential-oil.html

https://www.rodalesorganiclife.com/wellbeing/essential-oils-in-bath

https://www.organicfacts.net/health-benefits/essential-oils/health-benefits-of-bergamot-essential-oil.html

https://www.indigo-herbs.co.uk/natural-health-guide/benefits/clary-sage

https://www.organicfacts.net/health-benefits/essential-oils/health-benefits-of-frankincense-essential-oil.html

https://naha.org/explore-aromatherapy/about-aromatherapy/most-commonly-used-essential-oils

https://www.mayoclinic.org/drugs-supplements-tea-tree-oil/art-20364246

---

https://www.youngliving.com/en_US/products/roman-chamomile-essential-oil

https://www.aromaweb.com/essential-oils/roman-chamomile-oil.asp

Julia Lawless, *The Illustrated Encyclopedia of Essential Oils* (Rockport, MA: Element Books, 1995), 56-67.

https://draxe.com/ginger-essential-oil/

https://www.organicfacts.net/health-benefits/essential-oils/cypress-essential-oil.html

http://www.sustainablebabysteps.com/ylang-ylang-essen tial-oil.html

https://www.organicfacts.net/health-benefits/essential-oils/health-benefits-of-eucalyptus-essential-oil.html

https://www.youngliving.com/en_US/products/pepper mint-essential-oil

https://www.organicfacts.net/health-benefits/essential-oils/health-benefits-of-peppermint-oil.html

https://www.webmd.com/vitamins-supplements/ingredi entmono-719-lemongrass.aspx?activeingredientid=719&active ingredientname=lemongrass

https://www.organicfacts.net/health-benefits/essential-oils/wintergreen-essential-oil.html

https://www.livestrong.com/article/358387-spearmint-es sential-oil-benefits/

https://www.thefusionmodel.com/vanilla-essential-oil-ben efits-uses-and-side-effects/

https://www.dreamingearth.com/blog/make-your-own-aro matherapy-spritzers/

https://www.organicfacts.net/health-benefits/essential-oils/orange-essential-oil.html

https://www.organicfacts.net/health-benefits/essential-oils/vanilla-essential-oil.html

Tinctures & Supplements

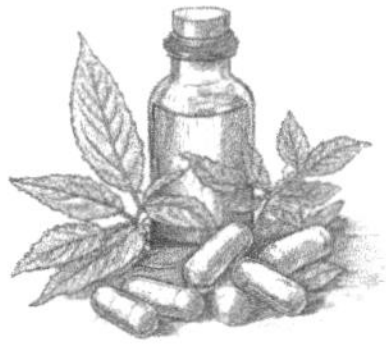

Tinctures are a type of herbal liquid extract made from various berries, or bark or leaves, or roots from one or more plants in vinegar or alcohol.

Tinctures can be purchased or made but one must be sure to follow the directions carefully. It is recommended that you purchase tinctures from a trusted source.

Commonly Used Tinctures:

- Elderberry
- Echinacea
- Turmeric

Elderberry (Sambucus nigra) has been said to have several beneficial properties.

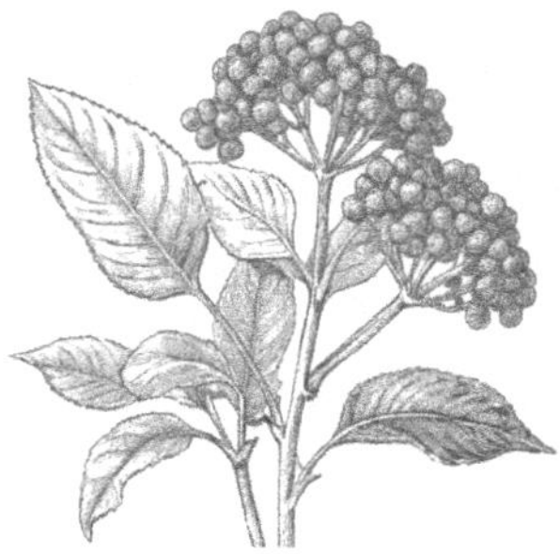

- Remove toxins
- Promote urine flow and bowel movements
- Colds and flu
- Heart Health
- Reduce inflammation in joints, tendons, ligaments, and muscles
- Rich in antioxidants

Precautions: Not intended for under 18 years old. May have adverse effects in some adults.

Echinacea (Echinacea purpurea) comes in various forms and supplements. Tinctures can be made or purchased from a trusted source.

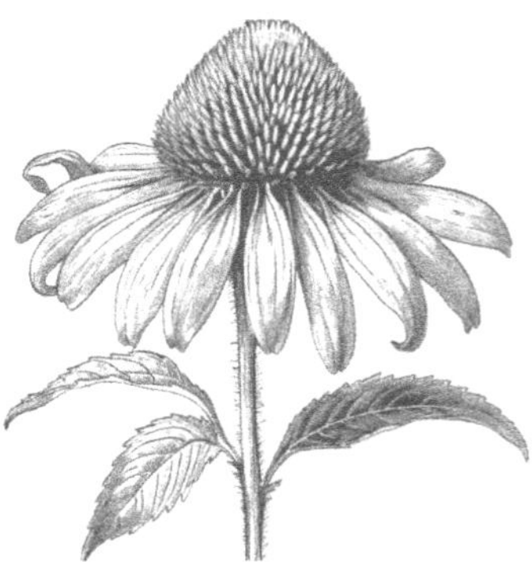

- Immune support
- Diabetes
- Anxiety
- Anti-inflammatory

Precautions: May be contraindicated in the presence of certain autoimmune disorders.

Turmeric (Curcuma longa) comes in various forms and supplements. Tinctures can be made or purchased from a trusted source.

- Anti-inflammatory
- Antioxidant
- Digestive

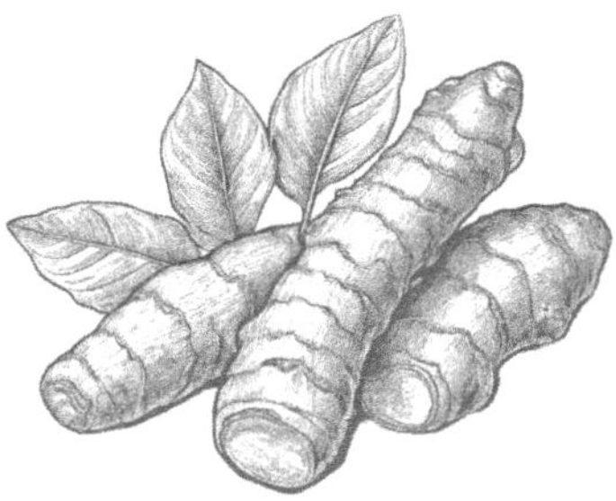

Precautions

Avoid with gallbladder issues, bleeding issues, and hormone related conditions.

End Notes:[1]

Healthy Super Foods

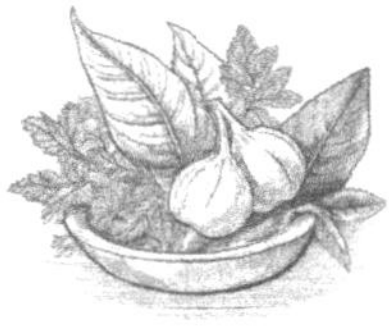

Although there are tons of healthy foods to consume in this book, we are focusing on some of the super healthy foods to add to dishes and some of the lesser-known foods along with suggested uses and benefits.

Food, Herbs, and Spices

There are many foods, herbs, and spices that are associated with possible health benefits. It is always best to consult with your healthcare provider and a nutritionist for guidance on your individual nutritional needs which vary based on age, genetics, and the presence of medical/health conditions. Generally, a healthy diet should include:

- Lean proteins
- Whole Grains
- Vegetables
- Fruits
- Water*
- Limit sugars and salts
- Focus on healthy fats

Apple Cider Vinegar

Vinegars are frequently touted as beneficial to one's health and apple cider vinegar has become very popular. It can be added to salads, water, and certain teas. It may also be dabbed on acne and other minor skin ailments. Depending on what you are hoping to achieve with the use of apple cider vinegar you should consult with your healthcare provider.

---

* consult with healthcare provider

Apple Cider Vinegar

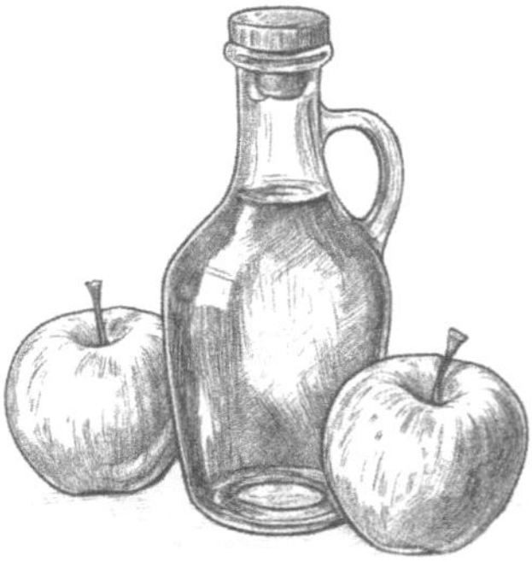

- May help to control blood sugar
- Weight loss
- Acne and mosquito bites
- Blood pressure
- Cholesterol

Precautions: Avoid taking full strength. It's better to dilute it. May irritate skin so only use in small amounts and check with your healthcare provider

Avocado

Avocado has many health benefits and can be added to salads and sandwiches.

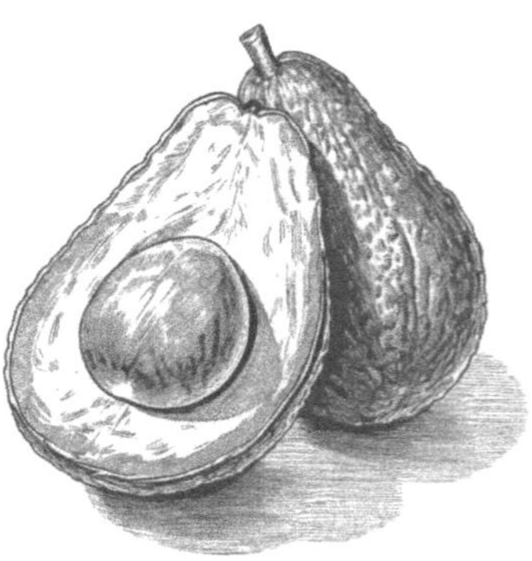

- Skin health
- Heart health
- Protects liver

- Eye health
- Morning sickness

Precautions: May cause headaches

Guacamole Recipe

Ingredients:

- 2 ripe avocados
- 1/4 cup of red onion
- 1/4 cup of chopped tomato
- 1/4 cup diced jalapeño
- 1 tbsp chopped cilantro
- 1 tsp of fresh lime choice
- Salt, and pepper to taste

Directions:

1. Cut avocados in half and scoop into a medium bowl
2. Add all ingredients and then mix to desired consistency
3. Serve with chips or spread on whole grain toast

Cucumbers

Cucumbers are fruits that have many benefits and contain Vitamins A, C, folic, and magnesium. They may be added to salads or water and are used to make pickles.

- Skin Care
- Puffy eyes
- May lower blood pressure
- Prevents constipation
- May reduce risk of kidney stones

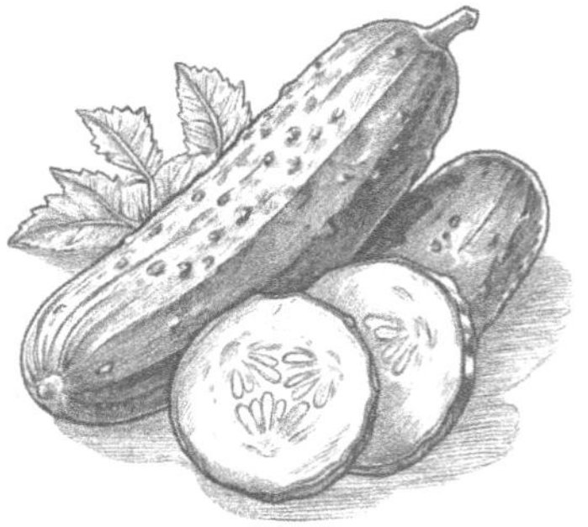

Lemons

Lemons are one of the citrus fruits that contain beneficial vitamins and minerals (e.g., Vitamins C, A, B6, E, zinc, iron, potassium, magnesium, and niacin) and antioxidant properties. It can be added to various foods and teas and even used topically.

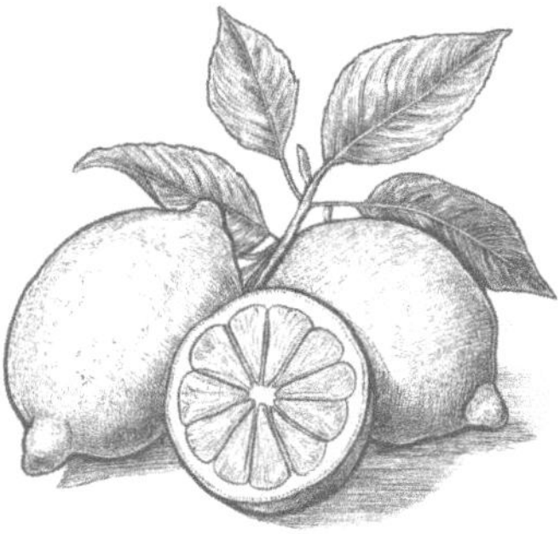

- Weight loss
- Indigestion
- Blood pressure control
- Constipation
- Skin care/ Bee stings
- Arthritis
- Toothaches
- Sore throats

Precautions: May cause migraines

Lemon Sore Throat Remedy

- Hot Tea
- 1 tsp lemon juice
- 1 tbsp of raw honey

Kale

Kale is a vegetable that is packed with vitamins A, B6, C, K, Manganese, Copper, Potassium, and Magnesium. It has been touted as one of the healthiest foods. Kale can be added to salads, smoothies, and soups. It can also be sautéed in olive oil and garlic.

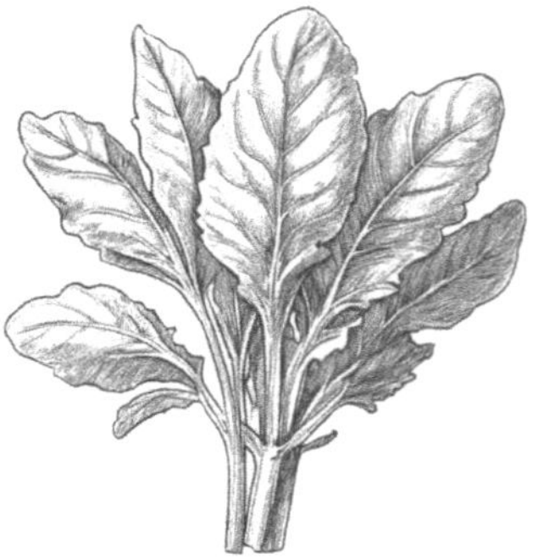

- Antioxidant
- Helps reduce cholesterol
- Cancer Fighting
- Eye health
- Weight Loss
- Great source of potassium
- High in Beta Carotene

Raw Honey

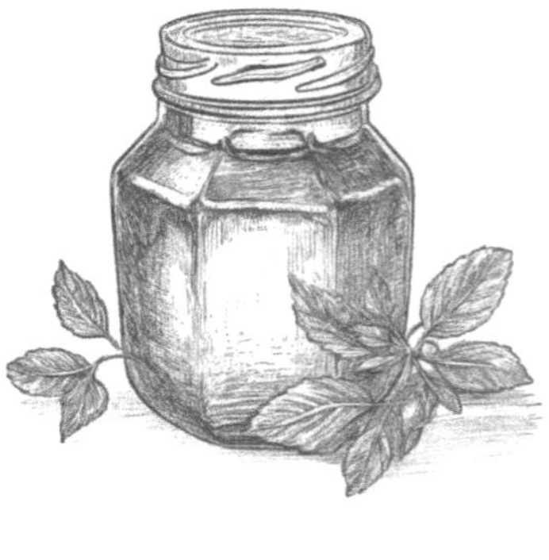

Raw honey is taken directly from the beehive and has many health benefits. It can be added to teas, oatmeal, or any foods you would like to sweeten.

- Antiviral/Antifungal
- Antioxidants

- Skin conditions
- Blood sugar
- Immune system
- Allergies

Precautions: Do not give regular or raw honey to children before consulting with your pediatrician. May cause food poisoning, allergies and in some cases intoxication.

Quinoa

Quinoa is a grain that is packed with proteins and nutrients, associated with many health benefits and is gluten-free.

- High fiber
- Controls blood sugar
- Metabolic health
- antioxidants

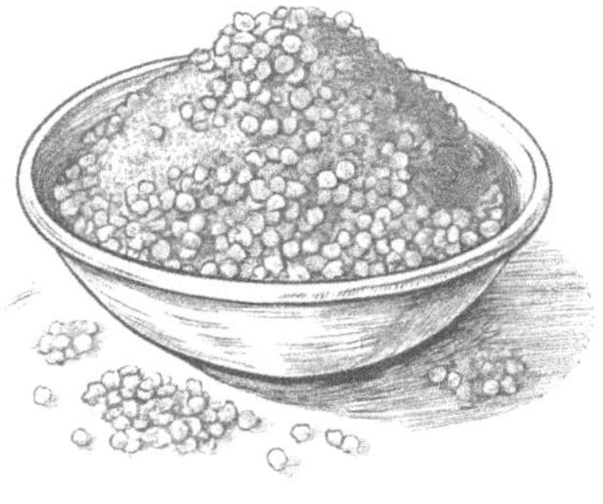

Precautions:

Discontinue if sensitivity develops, Discuss with healthcare provider if pregnant

Quinoa Recipe

Quinoa is cooked like rice, you can add veggies such as kale and sweet potatoes.

1. Mix 1 cup of quinoa (rinsed) and 2 cups of water or broth, and ¼ tsp salt
2. Bring to a boil and simmer for 15-20 minutes until water is absorbed

Tomatoes

Tomatoes are considered a vegetable and a fruit and are packed with all kinds of nutrients. There are many different types which can be used in a variety of recipes.

- Antioxidant
- Heart health
- Improve vision
- Skin care
- Helps to manage diabetes
- May prevent UTI's, gallstones

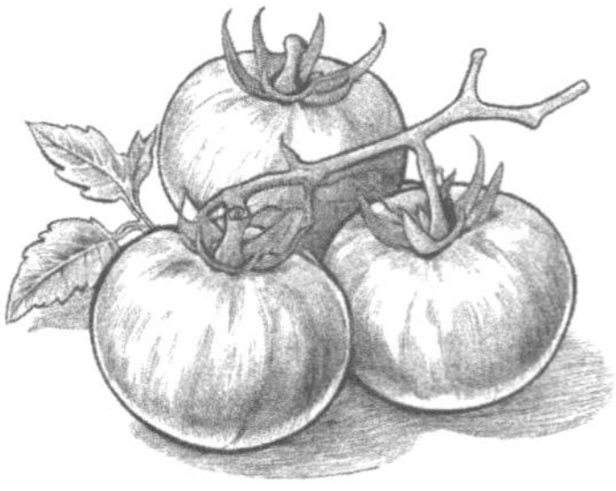

Reishi Mushrooms (Ganoderma lucidum and lingzhi)

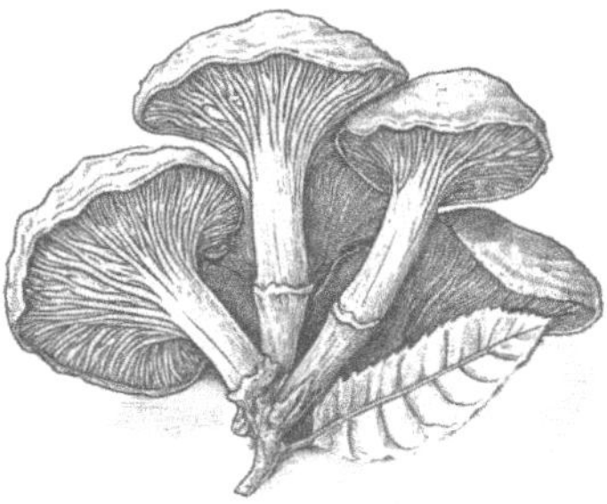

- Boosts immune system
- Anti-cancer
- Fatigue and depression
- Heart health
- Blood sugar control
- Antioxidant

Precautions: Avoid when breastfeeding, with hypotension, blood disorders, or undergoing surgery.

Acai berries (Euterpe oleracea, Euterpe badiocarpa)

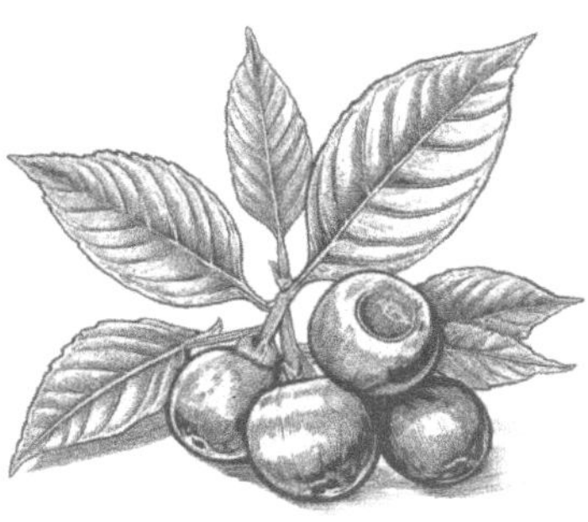

Acai berries are harvested from acai palm trees.

- Cognitive function

- Heart health
- Anti-cancer

Precautions: May affect MRI results. Check with the healthcare provider if pregnant or nursing. Avoid drinking unprocessed acai juice.

Flax Seeds (Linum usitatissimum)

Flax seeds have been used for hundreds of years and have many health benefits.

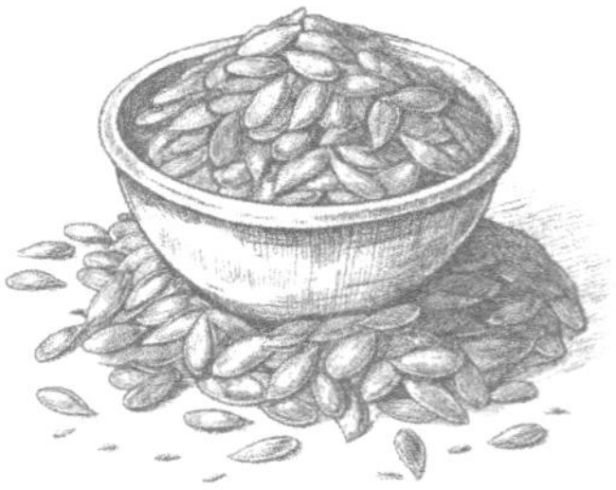

- Good source of nutrients and omega-3 fats and fiber
- Decrease cancer risk
- Lower blood sugar
- Improve cholesterol
- Lower blood pressure
- Weight control

Precautions: Limit to less than 5 tablespoons per day.

Chia Seeds

Chia seeds are a great source of fiber and omega 3.

- Weight loss
- Diabetes
- Diverticulosis
- Heart Health
- Digestion

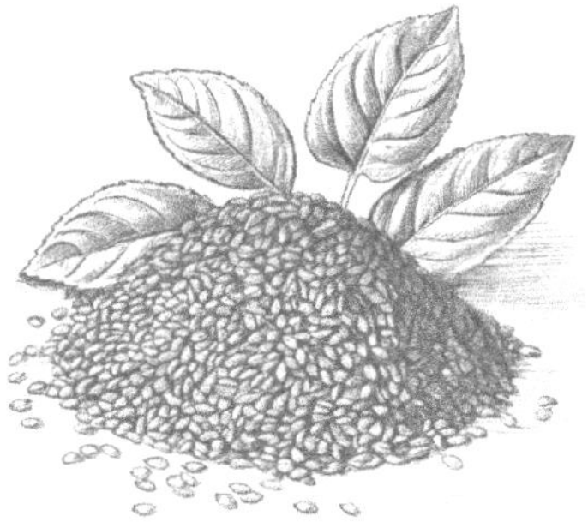

Precautions:

Avoid swallowing disorders and in young children.

Dragon Fruit (Hylocereus cactus)

Dragon fruit is high in antioxidants and high in fiber.

- Chronic disease
- Gut health
- Boost immune system
- Increase iron levels

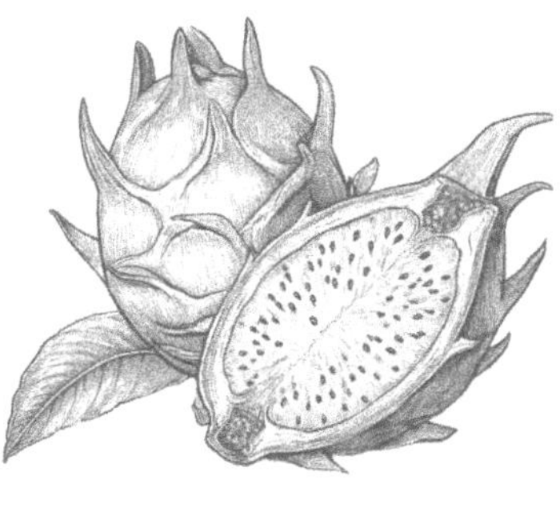

- Good source of magnesium

Precautions: May cause a severe allergic reaction.

Healthy Shakes/Smoothies

There are lots of ways to incorporate the healthy foods, herbs, and spices described in this book. Here is an example:

Berry Banana Kale Turmeric Smoothie

Ingredients: Skim milk or orange juice~ 8 Oz., 1/2 banana, 1/2 cup berries, 1 cup of Kale, 1/4 tsp of ground turmeric [1]

Supplements & Vitamins

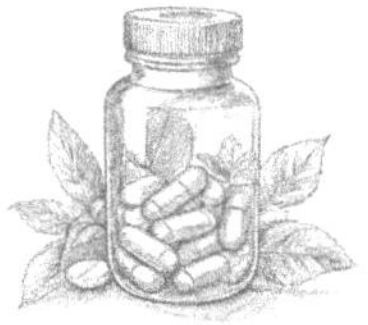

The use of probiotics, dietary supplements, and vitamins should also be considered in your health and wellness regimen.

Probiotics

Probiotics are live bacteria and yeast. Probiotics are often called "good" or "helpful" bacteria because they are intended to keep your gut healthy. It is important to note that additional research is required in this area.

Potential Benefits:

- Digestion
- Diarrhea

- Heart health
- Weight loss
- Immune health

Precautions: It is important to purchase quality products
1

Vitamins and Supplements

There are numerous vitamins and supplements that are touted to have positive effects on one's health. Although there is some evidence to support these claims, many have not been well-studied so it is important to discuss the use of vitamins and supplements with your healthcare provider. According to the National Institute of Health*"Because foods provide an array of nutrients and other components that have benefits for health, nutritional needs should be met primarily through foods. ... In some cases, fortified foods and dietary supplements are useful when it is not pos-

* (2021) The federal government's 2020–2025 Dietary Guidelines for Americans

sible otherwise to meet needs for one or more nutrients (e.g., during specific life stages such as pregnancy)."

Herbs and Spices

Herbs and spices are used to enhance the flavor of many foods and many also have health benefits. You may choose fresh or dried herbs.

There are many benefits associated with herbs and spices. We will provide an overview of some of the most common ones and recommend that you do your own research on the benefits and uses of your favorite herbs and spices. Planting your own herb garden on a deck, terrace, windowsill, or backyard is a great way to ensure you have plenty of fresh herbs on hand.

Cacao

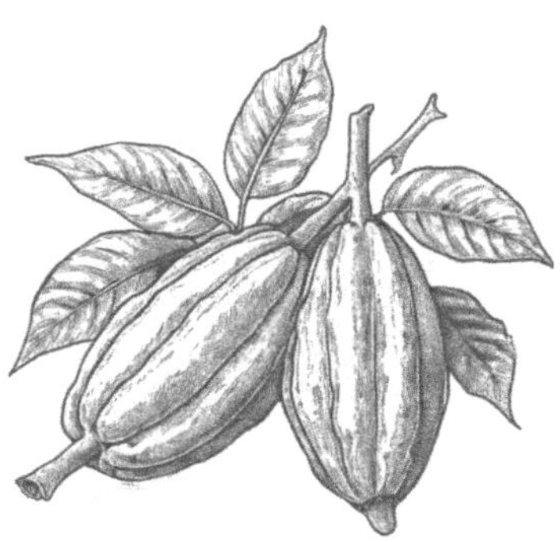

Raw cacao differs from cocoa and has numerous health benefits. It is a powerful antioxidant and rich in iron and magnesium.

Potential Benefits:

- Mood elevator/Antidepressant
- Improve memory
- Weight loss
- Skin care
- Lowers blood pressure

Precautions: Consult with a healthcare provider prior to use.

Cardamom

Cardamom is a spice that is thought to have numerous health benefits and contains magnesium, niacin, riboflavin, vitamin A and C, and calcium.

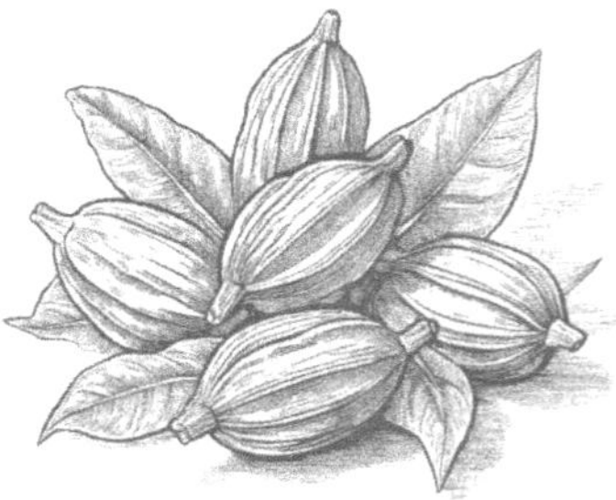

Potential Benefits:

- Heart health
- Nausea and vomiting
- Anti-depressant

- Heart health
- Prevents gastrointestinal disease

Precautions: Do not use during pregnancy

Cayenne Pepper

Cayenne peppers are packed with nutrients and antioxidants. They are hot and are used in many spicy dishes (peppers or powder)

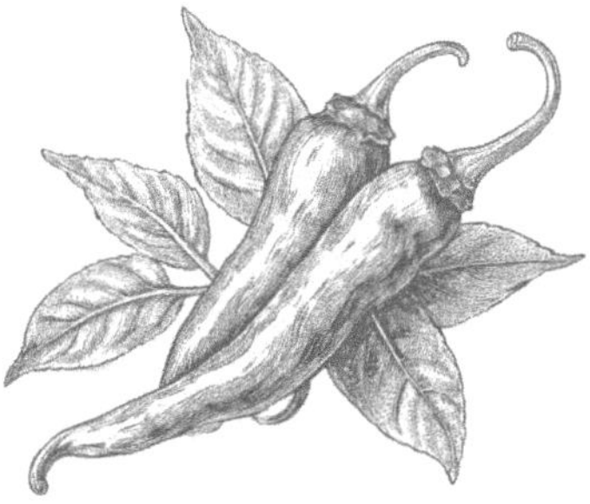

Potential Benefits:

- Boost metabolism and digestion
- Reduce hunger
- Lower blood pressure
- Pain relief (capsaicin cream)
- Psoriasis

Precautions: Check with Healthcare provider if taking blood thinners

Cinnamon

Cinnamon is made from the Cinnamomum tree and its use dates to ancient Egypt. It is best to use Ceylon cinnamon.

Potential Benefits:

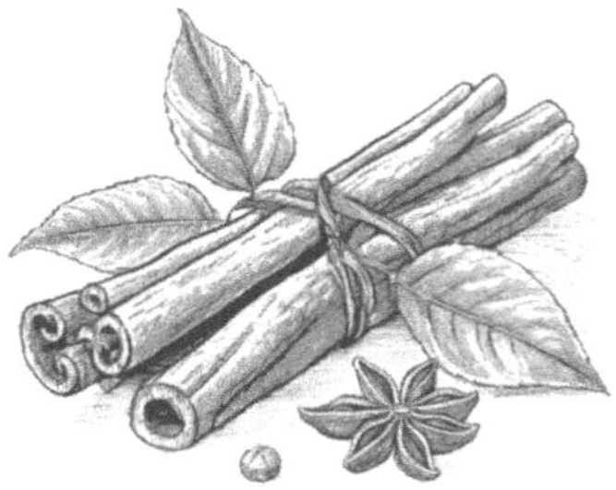

- Antioxidant
- Anti-inflammatory
- Lower risk of heart disease
- May lower blood sugar and decrease insulin resistance

Precautions: Too much Cassia cinnamon (most found in stores) can cause liver damage, mouth sores, and problems with breathing

Cucumbers

Cucumbers are fruits that are packed with nutrients and have several health benefits.

Potential benefits:

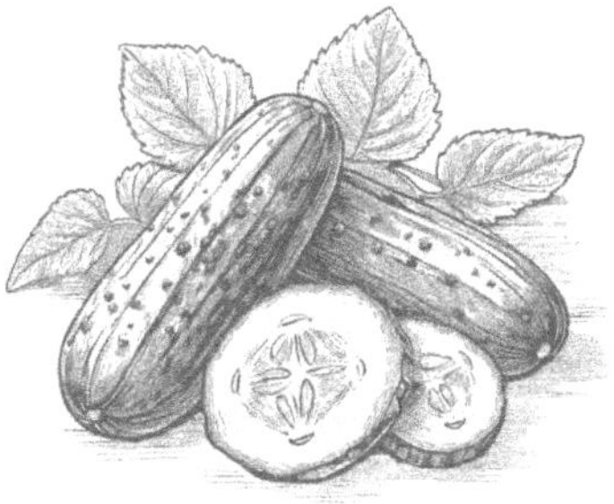

- Skin care
- Manage blood sugar
- Lower blood pressure
- Prevent constipation
- Prevent kidney stones

Precautions: May cause oral allergies

Fennel

Fennel is an herb used in cooking that is associated with many health benefits.

Potential benefits:

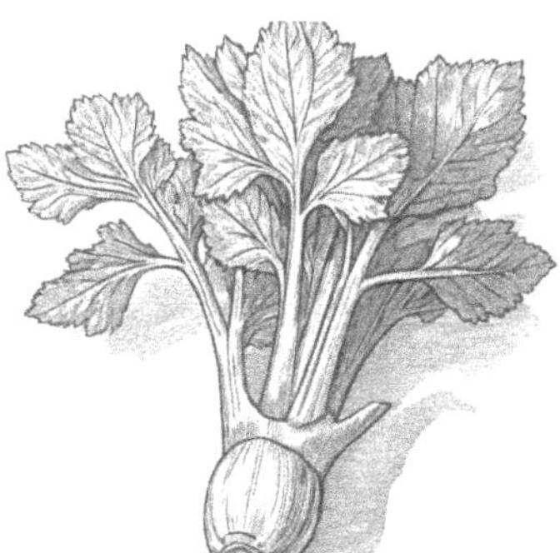

- Heartburn
- Gas and bloating
- Cough
- Colic (check with pediatrician
- Back-aches

Precautions: Check with healthcare provider if pregnant or nursing or bleeding disorders

Garlic

Garlic has been used for medicinal purposes and cooking and has many nutrients.

Potential benefits:

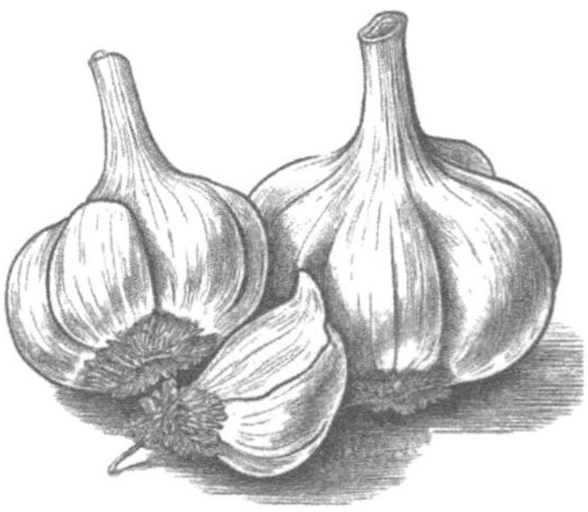

- Lowers blood pressure
- Cold remedy
- Bone health
- Dementia
- May lower cholesterol

Precautions: May irritate the stomach or cause bleeding.

Ginger

Ginger is a spice that is used in many recipes and is known to have many health benefits.

Potential benefits:

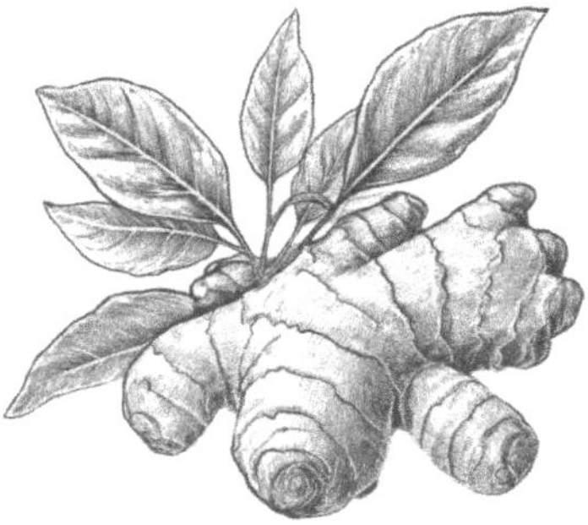

- Treat Nausea
- Anti-inflammatory and pain relief
- My lower blood sugar
- Improve heart health
- Indigestion

Precautions: Pregnant, Heart Disease, Diabetes

Parsley

Parsley is an herb that has been used for thousands of years, contains many nutrients, and is used in cooking and as a garnish.

Potential benefits:

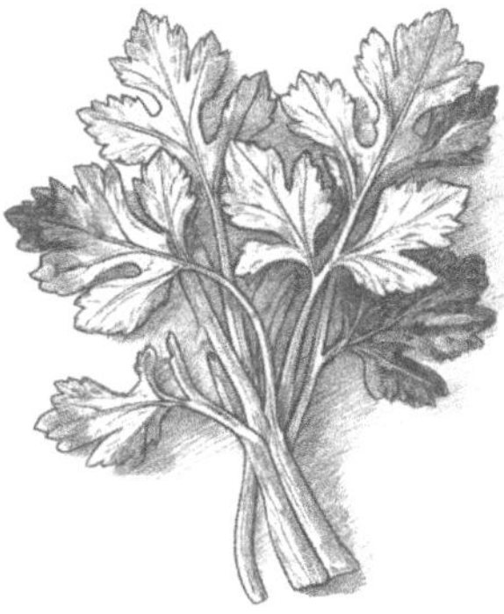

- May decrease blood sugar
- Anti-inflammatory
- Improves immune system

- Improves digestion
- Diuretic

Precautions: Check with healthcare provider

Rosemary

Rosemary is an herb that is used to enhance the flavor of many foods and is associated with several health benefits.

Potential benefits:

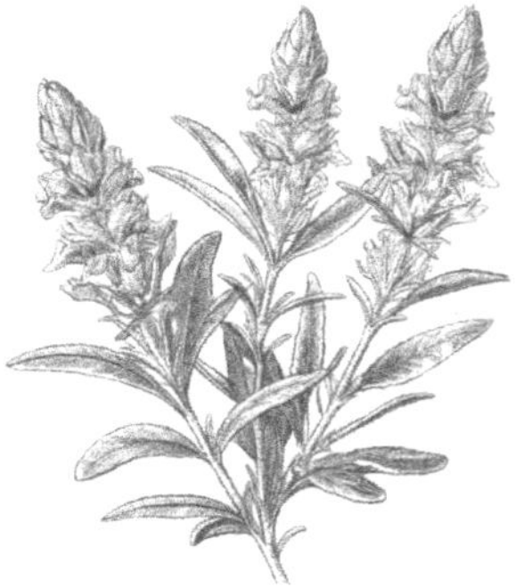

- Stress
- Helps immunity system
- Fresh breath
- Pain relief

Precautions: Do not use it if you have a seizure disorder, allergic to aspirin, or bleeding.

Sage

Sage is an herb that has many medicinal properties and has been used for thousands of years.

Potential benefits:

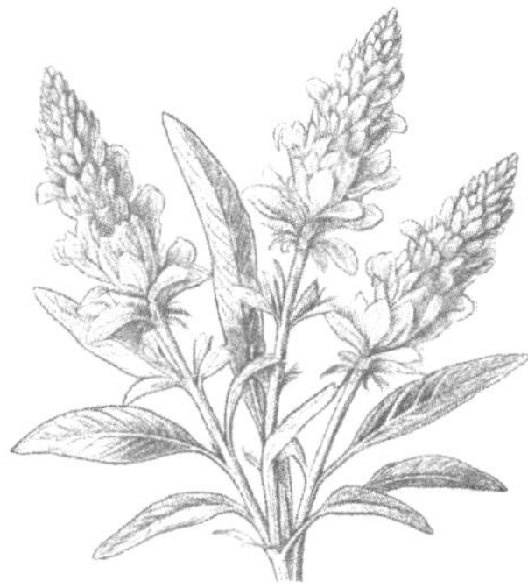

- Treats inflammation
- Skin care
- Digestive aid
- Bone health
- Diabetes management

Precautions: May cause allergic reaction

Turmeric

Turmeric is a spice that is often used in Asian dishes and has several health benefits.

Potential benefits:

- Digestion/Heartburn
- Arthritis/Pain/Headaches
- Irritable bowel disease/syndrome

- Lung infections/ Colds
- Alzheimer's disease

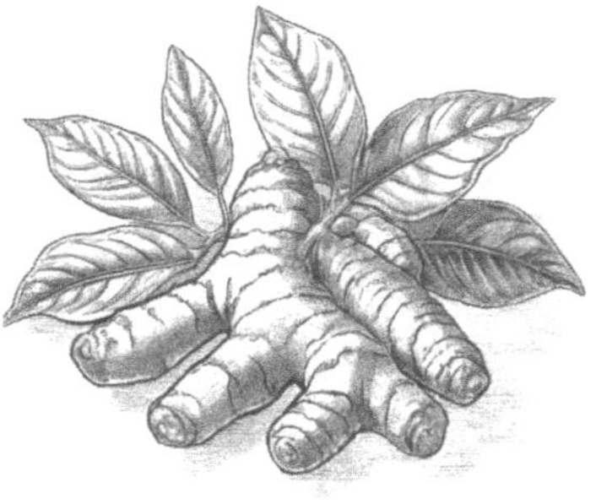

Precautions: Use with caution if pregnant

Nourishing One's Mind

Journaling and Cognitive-Behavioral Therapy

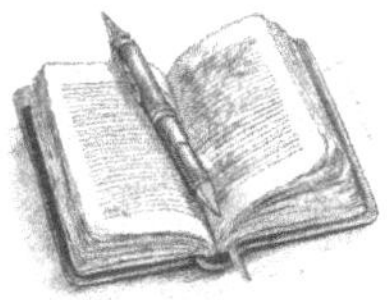

We are living in extremely stressful times, and it is important to consider what types of support you need, which may vary at different times during your life.

Some things can be done individually and independently such as journaling and others, such as various psychological and behavioral therapy require a trained professional who can offer these types of support. These may include Psychoanalysis, Psychotherapy, Cognitive Behavioral Therapy, and Biotherapy.

Journaling

Journaling provides many benefits and there are many ways one can journal. The practice can be formal or informal. Journaling involves writing your thoughts, feelings, and experiences. You may write in a journal or notebook or on your computer.

Reflective journaling requires one to read their journal entries and reflect on them. This can be a way of "letting go" of negative emotions, or for reinforcing positive experiences.

There is a practice called "Schedule Your Worry Time" where you set aside time to worry about what you need to get done and plan for it, instead of allowing these worries to follow you around all day.[1]

Journaling Exemplar

By John Hunt

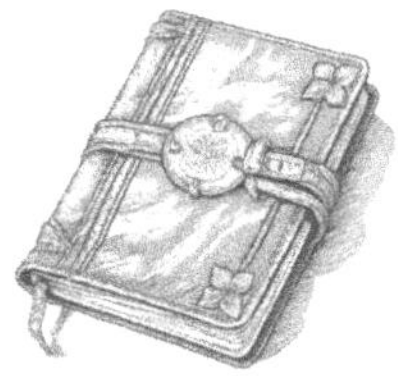

Journaling, while being among the simplest self-care practices, is also among the most beneficial. Journaling is a form of self-expression, perhaps among one of the most direct forms of it, in which you simply write about parts of your day. Whether your journal entries focus ongoing into detail about a specific event, or just writing about your current emotions, it can have plenty of benefits. You may choose to write on your computer or purchase a special notebook or journal.

To list a few:

- Consistently writing about yourself can make you more mindful of your actions. With increased mindfulness, comes increased awareness of our minds, and with increased awareness comes increased control over our thoughts and emotions.
- While a daily journal of your events will obviously help you remember parts of your life, the act of recalling memories from the day and writing them down can improve our ability to remember and recall information.
- Writing troubling events and emotions have helped relieve people from the stress they experience.

Yoga & Acupuncture

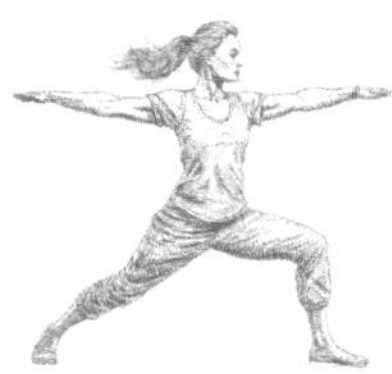

Alternative and Complementary healing modalities have become quite popular. Some you can learn how to do at home and others need to be done by a trained professional.

Yoga

Yoga (yuj-to unite) is an ancient practice that uses breathing(pranayama), meditation, and various stretching and yoga poses that date back over 5,000 years. Although you can teach yourself or watch videos, attending some formal classes is very helpful. You should check with your healthcare provider before engaging in Yoga and/or other activities discussed in this book.

Potential benefits:

- Improves flexibility
- Improves posture
- Bone health
- Lowers blood pressure and blood sugar
- Boosts immune system
- Inner strength

Acupuncture/Acupressure/Cupping/ Coining/ Herbal Medicine

Traditional Chinese Medicine includes acupuncture and acupressure, cupping, coining, use of herbs, diet, and mind/body healing.

Acupuncture involves insertion of small needles on the various meridians in the body and acupressure is similar but does not use needles. The goal of acupuncture or acupressure is to restore the balance of energy in the body. It is very important to visit a licensed/certified practitioner.

Acupuncture/Acupressure

Potential benefits:

- Pain management
- Depression
- Nausea
- Migraines
- Promotes well-being
- Parkinson's disease

Precautions: Bleeding disorders

Complimentary Therapy

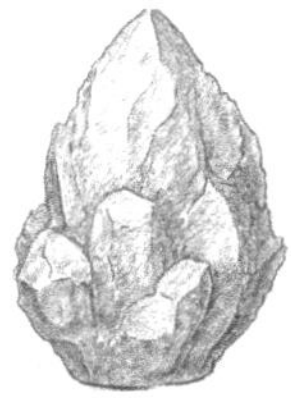

Cryotherapy

Cryotherapy dates back to ancient times and has been widely used particularly to reduce inflammation. Recently it has been used as Whole body cryotherapy to promote physical and mental well-being. WBC is a kind of cryogenic therapy where the entire body is exposed to very cold temperatures for a short time. You are placed in a tank where the temperature may exceed -200 degrees Fahrenheit for 2-4 minutes. Some posit that it can help to treat pain, depression, and fibromyalgia although It is not FDA approved and has not been well studied. Furthermore, the American Academy of Dermatology Association points out that it may be harmful to the skin and cause frostbite and rashes. They do not recommend its use and caution to consult with one's healthcare provider before using. *

Infrared Sauna

Infrared saunas use infrared lights to provide various health benefits. Unlike a traditional heated sauna the temperature are lower and the infrared lights also have an electromagnetic effect. Research has demonstrated a correlation with improved heart health, lower blood pressure, pain relief, improved circulation, and sleep, and preventing the common cold. It should not be used in patients with Multiple Sclerosis, when your sick, or during pregnancy, and while trying to conceive. †

* https://www.aad.org/public/cosmetic/safety/cryotherapy https://www.webmd.com/pain-management/what-is-whole-body-cryorapy

† https://health.clevelandclinic.org/infrared-sauna-benefits

Salt Rooms/Caves and Salt Lamps

Salt rooms or caves deliver a dry salt experience and are associated with multiple health benefits. There are two types of salt rooms, one is considered "Active" for halotherapy where machines break apart the salt allowing them to be exposed to the skin and inhaled. The other type is a "Passive" room which is filled with Himalayan salt and a meditative experience.

Potential benefits:

- Improved breathing
- Fights Infections
- Healthier skin
- Stress reduction

Potential risks include: Coughing, Lack of standardization regarding salt therapy, Lack of evidence

Salt Lamps

Himalayan salt lamps are associated with several benefits although there is very little evidence to support the claims. They are different size crystals carved from amber-colored rock salt, hollowed out to fit a lightbulb inside.

Potential benefits:

- Improve sleep
- Improve breathing
- Help with Asthma and allergies
- Decreased in anxiety and depression (studies have been one on rats and mice which have shown a correlation. Further investigation is warranted)*

* https://health.clevelandclinic.org/salt-cave-benefits

Hypnotherapy

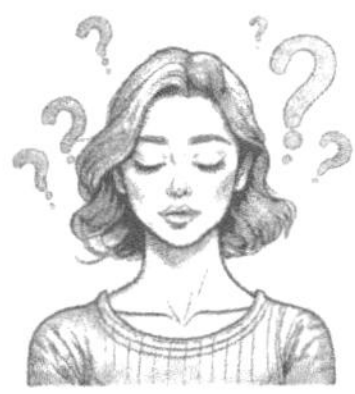

The National Society of Clinical Hypnosis states that hypnosis has been used for many years and helps an individual enter a natural state where they can enter a state of consciousness and focused attention. It usually involves the person going into a trance-like state where they are still aware, but their minds are open to suggestions. It's important to visit an experienced provider.

Hypnotherapy

Potential Benefits:

- Weight loss

- Treat addictions
- Pain management
- Stress reduction
- Improved sleep
- Treat anxiety and depression

Precautions: Check with healthcare provider in presence of mental illness

Sleep Habits

Our bodies need to rest and getting a good night's sleep helps our physical, mental, and emotional well-being.

Sleep Hygiene Tips:

- Avoid caffeine at night
- Exercise during the day
- Create a relaxing space
- Sleep in a darkened room
- Establish a regular bedtime
- Avoid eating heavy food at night

Meditation

By Jaime Hunt

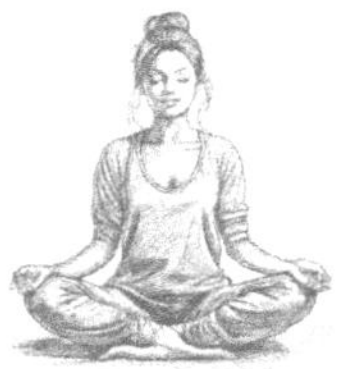

At times, one's thought process may be challenged but meditating is a gateway to find that freedom. Meditation is about grounding yourself and finding the center of your body and soul. You must feel at peace within both. We often tend to question ourselves, including the decisions we make. Meditation can give you clear insight and help you seek the answers you are looking for.

Potential Benefits:

- Stress reliever
- Happiness within oneself
- Better reactions to situations

- Calm sense of being
- Anti-depressant

Precautions: May become addicted to finding pure joy.

There are many ways to meditate and a plethora of resources available online. This is one that I do daily.

5 Easy Steps for Meditating:

Step 1: Find a calm/ tranquil place. Can be wherever you feel 'at peace' with minimal distractions.
Step 2: Find a comfortable seated position or lay down if you prefer. You want to find a space where you're able to have an even blood flow throughout the entire body.
Step 3: Try your best to clear all the thoughts from your mind. Use the space around you like storage boxes. Physically place each thought into an imaginary box

around you until you no longer have a thought.

Step 4: Now that you have cleared your mind and found that safe place, begin to take deep breaths in and out using your diaphragm. Remember, you are in control of your body and your thoughts. No one can harm you while you are meditating.

Step 5: You may stay in this meditative state for as long as you wish. You've fulfilled all the necessary steps to meditation. There is no time limit on how long you should meditate. You should take as long as you need.

Deep Breathing Exercises

Deep breathing exercises are simple to do and help one relax. They are also used in meditation and hypnosis. This is one example, however there are many types of deep breathing exercises you can learn and practice.

Steps:

- Get comfortable
- Close eyes or look downwards
- Inhale deeply
- Exhale slowly
- Repeat 3-6 times
- Do this throughout the day as often as you need

Sudarshan kriya yoga (SKY)

There are four main SKY breathing techniques:

- "Om" is chanted three times during exhalation.
- Bhastrika ("Bellow Breath") breathing requires 30 breaths per minute of rapid inhalation with forceful exhalation.
- Ujjayi ("Victorious Breath") is a slow breathing technique to promote calmness and alertness
- Sudarshan Kriya is rhythmic breathing with varying cycles of

breathing*

* Zope SA, Zope RA. Sudarshan kriya yoga: Breathing for health. Int J Yoga. 2013 Jan;6(1):4-10. doi: 10.4103/0973-6131.105935. PMID: 23440614; PMCID: PMC3573542.

Nourishing One's Spirit

Therapeutic Touch/Reiki

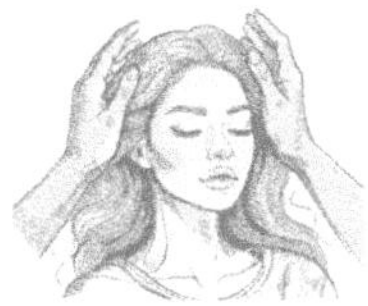

Therapeutic Touch is an alternative healing modality that was developed in the 1970's by Delores Krieger and Dora Kunz and is based on laying on of hands from ancient times. Unlike Reiki, the practitioner does not touch the patient. The process involves several steps that have some variability. At the beginning of the session the practitioner centers themselves and makes a silent intention for using energy in a positive manner. It is also important to protect oneself from potential negative energy and one might visualize themselves protected by a white light. The patient sits or lies in a comfortable position and might be guided to do a brief meditation. Next an assessment of the energy fields in proximity (1-2 inches above) to the patient is done. The practitioner then used their hands and energy to unruffle any blocked energy fields noted during the assessment phase. The final step is to do a head-to-toe rebalancing of the energy field.

According to the Therapeutic Touch International Association *therapeutic touch restores balance in mind, body, and spirit through the use of universal energy. You will need to find a trained practitioner.

Therapeutic Touch Possible Benefits:

- Promotes overall health and well-being
- Treats pain and anxiety
- Treats cancer related nausea, vomiting, weakness, and fatigue

Precautions: Avoid during pregnancy

* (2018)

Reiki

Reiki is like Therapeutic Touch regarding energy and restoring balance. However, it's a Japanese technique and the practitioner may lay their hands on the person's body.

Potential Benefits:

- Stress reduction
- Well-being
- Pain management
- Emotional well-being
- May improve immune system

Massage

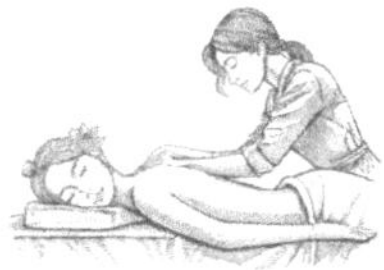

Massages are very beneficial and incorporate deep or light massage and manipulation of various muscles and tissues. You can learn how to self-massage, too. According to the Mayo Clinic there are several types of massages:

- Sports massage
- Deep tissue massage
- Trigger point massage
- Swedish massage

Potential benefits:

- Decreased stress

- Pain management
- Decreased anxiety
- Treat headaches
- Treat sports injuries (muscle and tissue)

Precautions:

Be sure to use a certified/licensed and experienced practitioner and share your comfort level.

Folk/ Traditional Medicine

Exemplars Around the Globe

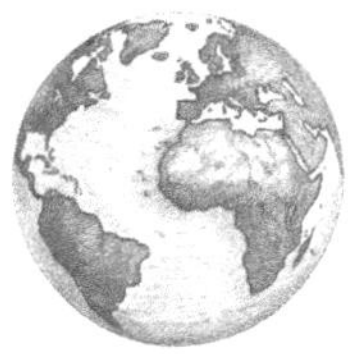

Many of the practices discussed in this book have roots in folk healing and some are unique to specific cultures.Many cultures use folk medicine that has been in existence for many years. It is a combination of medicine, spirituality, herbal, and traditional therapies. It is interesting to explore your family history and learn about folk practices that have been handed down through the generations. Your family may have passed down some of these practices to you. *

* https://www.who.int/news-room/feature-stories/detail/traditional-medicine-has-a-long-history-of-contributing-to-conventional-medicine-and-continues-to-hold-promise

Jamaica

In Jamaican Folk Medicine illness can be classified as the occult, spiritual, or natural. The cause dictates the treatment.

Common healers:

- Bush doctor (aka bush man) heals with herbs and has extensive knowledge of herbs
- Nanna or lay midwife uses various herbs to support childbirth

Bush medicine includes bush teas, bush baths, root tonic, and poultices.*

Herbs for ailments

- Stomach ailments: cola acuminato or bichy tree.
- Earaches: Cleome gynandra or bastard mustard

---

* https://ebookcentral.proquest.com/lib/adelphi/reader.action?docID=4388446&ppg=1

Ireland

In ancient Ireland a chamomile, a sprig of lavender or mint tied around the wrist to treat an upset stomach. And nettles were used to treat arthritis pain. They would make a soup with the nettles or ground them up and place them on the affected areas. Wounds were treated with honey and skin conditions were treated with seawood. *

Italy

Sage is used as an anti-bacterial, astringent, and anti-fungal. Olive is used in cooking and to treat minor burns. White bread is used for stomach acid. A warm onion can treat earaches. †

---

* https://irishfolktours.com/irish-folk-remedies/

† Romeo N, Gallo O, Tagarelli G. From Disease to Holiness: Religious-based health remedies of Italian folk medicine (XIX-XX century). J Ethnobiol Ethnomed. 2015 Jun 6;11:50. doi: 10.1186/s13002-015-0037-z. PMID: 26048412; PMCID: PMC4468812.

Sumeria, Egypt, and Greece

The Sumerians and Egyptians used the bark from the willow tree for pain relief and inflammation. The Greeks also used it for fevers and to reduce the pain of childbirth. Interestingly, willow bark is the basis of aspirin. Interestingly, a chemist named Felix Hoffman synthesized aspirin in 1897 and it improved the lives of millions of people.

Mexico and Latin America

The "hot-cold syndrome" is a belief that some foods cause "cold disorders" and some cause "hot disorders", An example of illnesses related to cold entering the body are colds, stomach cramps, pain, and tuberculosis. An example of illnesses related to an overabundance of heat entering the body are sore throat, dysentery, kidney ailments, and sore eyes. A pregnant woman has an unusually warm body during the entire course. A woman who is pregnant usually has a warm body so she should avoid cold foods.*

* Currier, Richard L. "THE HOT-COLD SYNDROME

Activities and Exercise

Engaging in various activities can be a fun way to decrease stress and improve well-being. The important thing is to find something that makes you happy. Exercise is a great way to get healthy and stay healthy. There are many activities you can do, but always check with your healthcare provider and find something you enjoy, such as:

- Dancing (formal or freestyle)
- Tae-Kwon-do
- Tae-Chi
- Swimming
- Walking/Hiking/Cycling
- Exercise (find something you love)
- Sports (so many options)
- Music (listening or learning to play an instrument)
- Reading (book clubs are fun)

AND SYMBOLIC BALNCE IN MEXICAN AND SPANISH -AMERICAN FOLK MEDICINE." *Ethnology* 5.3 (1966): 251–263. Print

- Hobbies (painting, gardening, knitting, cooking, photography, etc.

These are just a few examples of ways to stay active and engaged. The key is to find something you enjoy and nourish your mind, body, and spirit.

Cycling: An Exemplar

By Brian Hunt

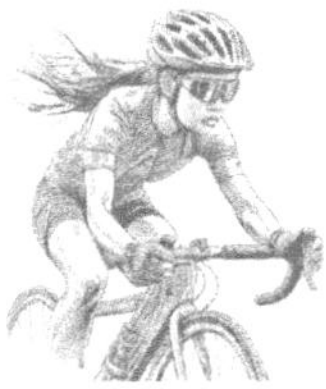

When I was growing up, I was fortunate enough to grow up on a block where there were tons of kids my age. As the years went on, we would play all the usual games that children would play.

Wiffle Ball, tag, football, basketball, you name it. As we grew up a bit more, we all started to take up BMX bikes. As a kid, the ultimate freedom that you could find was via a bicycle. I would wake up every summer morning and ride my bike with my friends from sunup to sundown. Locations that seemed far away and unreachable if not for a ride from a parent were now only a quick bike ride away. We would travel to local parks, friend's houses, candy stores, and when we were hungry, we would fuel up on pizza. Growing up in the Bronx, there was no shortage of amazing Pizzerias to indulge in. Even better, basically all the pizza shop owners were from the neighborhood, so they were always friendly to us and would let us store our bikes in a secure spot within their shop. As the years went on, cycling always held a special place in my heart. However, once I started high school, I noticed that I had less and less time for cycling as I was now in school all morning and started working every afternoon. Needless to say, my day was pretty much booked with everything except for cycling! During high school, I had time for school, work, and when I would get home; I would play video games for the rest of the night. As such, it wasn't long before I started to gain some weight and was living an unhealthy lifestyle. From freshman year through senior year, I would only ride my bike here and there. I knew that I wanted to get back into it, but it was difficult to change my lifestyle at that point. Difficult, but not impossible! During the summer of senior year when I was transitioning into college, I decided to take cycling back up, and boy I'm happy I did. Over the summer I would ride 3-5 times a week, along with going to the gym. It wasn't long before I noticed the pounds started to drop and my fitness level increased. In addition to that, I found myself staying away from junk food and playing less and less video games. The beauty of cycling is that you can just throw your leg over a bike and ride wherever, however long you'd like. Fast forward a few years and I now cycle anywhere from 150-200 miles a week. Cycling has opened a whole new world of fitness, friendship, and exploration. Throughout the years I've met hundreds of people who have a similar story to me. The common factor in all our stories is that we cycle because it's our passion, but also because it's undoubtedly one of the most fun and effective forms of exercise. Difficult, but not impossible!

Being a huge advocate for cycling, I've been able to convert many of my friends and family members into cyclists as well. Friends who used to be runners, basketball, baseball, football players, and general exercise enthusiasts can all find something to love in the sport of cycling. So why start cycling you ask? I'll use the old cliché, why not? The health benefits of cycling have been documented everywhere from Wikipedia to top medical journals. There is no age limit, weight restriction, or required fitness level to start! My advice to you is to head to your local bike shop and ask for a bike fitting and some suggestions on a beginner bike. Having worked in a bike shop in the past, I may be biased, but I can guarantee that bike shop employees are some of the friendliest and most helpful people on the planet! Don't want to spend the money on a new bike if you're unsure of the sport? You can always try and find a used bike on a site like eBay or Craigslist, or perhaps borrow one from a friend! Once you have your trusty bike, what should you do next? Simple, go on a ride! A simple search on the internet will unlock an entire network of bicycle trails, preferred routes, and commonly traveled roads to get you started. Alternatively, if you're the kind of person who likes to head out and explore, feel free! Some of the most enjoyable rides I've ever been on were the ones in which I headed out on an unspecified road for as long as I wanted to. Then, when you're ready to turn around, simply plug in your home address to your GPS enabled Smartphone and let it guide you home! What's more, Google Maps contains a "bike route" feature, which will have you on the best bike route possible. The only danger with cycling is just how addicting it can be! With each ride you'll begin to build a base fitness level. As you continue cycling, you'll notice that you'll be able to travel further distances and a faster speed without fatiguing as quickly as you would when you started. Soon, 10-mile rides will turn into 20 – 30-mile rides. You'll begin to have a new set of "cycling" friends who share your passion for the sport as well. The best part? While all of this is going on and you're out there having fun, you're also whipping yourself into excellent shape. Cycling will have you shedding pounds, improving your cardiovascular system, and building lean muscle. A few common phrases we use in the cycling world are "outside is free" and "Why Cycle over Driving? Cycling runs on fat, saves money" Driving runs on money, makes you fat". So do yourself a favor and purchase/borrow/ or rent a bicycle! I guarantee you'll be smiling as you take in the beautiful scenery along routes that were previously inaccessible without the use of a bike.

Lastly, I'll leave you with a few words of ad-

vice; always have fun, always lookout for your fellow cyclists, and always wear a helmet!!

Ayurveda/Ayurvedic Medicine

Ayurveda is a practice that is over 3000 years old. The focus is on health promotion and balance between the mind, body, and spirit. It uses the elements of fire, water, air, earth, and space and each one relates to one of three doshas (life force energies) in the body. If you wish to explore this practice it is best to see an Ayurvedic Healthcare Practitioner.

Homeopathy

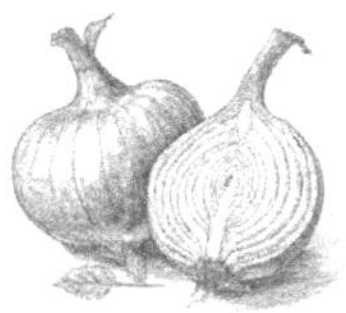

Homeopathy works on the premise that the body can heal itself. It was developed in the late 1700's. Homeopaths use small doses of plants and minerals to stimulate the healing process. In minuscule doses they are safe, but many can be toxic in higher doses, so it is best to consult with a Homeopathic Practitioner. The premise is that something that causes symptoms may treat certain conditions in very minuscule doses. Homeopaths use a process called "potentization" by adding water or alcohol to greatly weaken the substance. An example is the use of red onions for allergies because they make one's eyes water.

Complementary Therapy

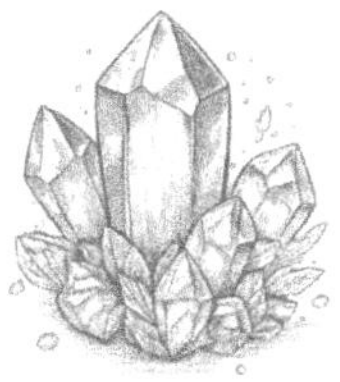

Crystal and Healing Powers

Crystals are considered by some to have protective and healing properties. Below is a small list of stones and properties. Some gemstones are used in Chakra cleansing which can help to restore balance in the body. A Chakra cleansing can be done with a practitioner or on your own. There are specific steps and does require meditation and focus on each chakra. There are 7 chakras in the body which are considered energy centers within the body. In Sanskrit chakras (wheels) are related to energy in the body that are influenced by colors and vibrations which correlate with spiritual well-being.

The seven main chakras and related colors and an example of related foods and gemstones are:

- Crown chakra- Sahasrara
    - (top of head)
    - white/purple
    - sage
    - clear quartz
- Third eye chakra - Ajna
    - (in between eyebrows)
    - indigo/violet
    - purple foods
    - amethyst
- Throat chakra - Vishuddha
    - (shoulder and neck areas)
    - blue
    - blueberries
    - lapis lazuli
- Heart chakra - Anahata
    - (center of chest)
    - pink
    - leafy greens

    - rose quartz
- Solar plexus chakra - Manipura
    - (belly button area)
    - yellow
    - complex carbs
    - tiger's eye
- Sacral chakra - Svadhisthana
    - (navel region)
    - orange
    - mangos
    - orange calcite
- Root chakra - Muladhara
    - (base of spine)
    - red
    - root vegetables
    - obsidian

You can read more about the chakras and how to do a cleanse on this website: https://consciousitems.com/blogs/practice/chakra-cleansing

- Rose Quartz: Circulation, Heart Chakra
- Quartz: Immune system All Chakras

- Citrine: Digestion, Crown and Solar Chakras
- Amethyst: Stress Reduction, Crown Chakra
- Golden Topaz: Overcoming nervous exhaustion
- Lapiz Lazuli: Migraines, Calming energy
- Blue Lace Agate: Nervous system. Calming effect
- Blood Stone: Sleep and Lymphatic stimulation Base and Heart Chakra
- Angelite: Grief and Emotional Pain
- Amber: Stress Reduction

Pets and Pet Therapy

Pets are known to be beneficial to your health. According to the CDC* pets provide an opportunity to exercise and socialize and can help to lower blood pressure, decrease blood sugar, triglycerides, and help to decrease loneliness.

Pet therapy is becoming more popular and

* (2019)

involves pet assisted therapy. Pet therapy is used to help with blood pressure, cancer, and mental health disorders.

Animal assisted activities are geared towards support and may include hospital or healthcare visits. For example, animals (dogs, rabbits, horses, and other animals) can be used in oncology units and help decrease pain, and anxiety during treatments. There are safety guidelines that must be followed but they have been beneficial.[1]

Weighted Blankets

Weighted blankets have become very popular and are available in different weights (5 -30 pounds). They can mimic a technique called deep pressure stimulation.

Potential benefits:

- Decreased stress
- Sleep Aid
- Decreased Anxiety

Some studies have found that this may benefit individuals with:

- Autism
- ADHD
- Sleep Disorders
- Pain

The use of art, dance, music, and imagery has many potential health benefits such as decreased anxiety, stress, depression, and improved quality of life.[2]

Music Therapy/Drumming

Music therapy involves the use of different types of music and can be used with or without a therapist individually or in a group setting. It includes listening to music, playing an instrument, singing, and discussing music. Studies have shown that music therapy as an adjuvant can help to decrease pain, nausea, and vomiting. It also helps patients to cope physically and mentally with their diagnosis.

Music has been enjoyed by many individuals

throughout the years and many cultures and religions have music that is unique and special. The benefits of music therapy have been documented for nearly a century although further study is required. Recently drumming has gained attention and a recent study demonstrated the positive effects it has on depression and anxiety and social resilience. Drumming is usually done in a group and may have a leader and be very structured but can also be done individually to one's own rhythm.

Art Therapy

Art therapists guide patients in the use of various artistic mediums such as photos, sculpture, drawings, and paintings to help them express their feelings. It is considered a body-mind therapy and is often used with cancer patients and may result in better quality of life and improved mood.

Dance Therapy

Dance therapy uses a variety of body movements which can help to reduce stress, anxiety, improve self-esteem and well-being, and decrease depression. The physical activity required in dance therapy increases the release of endorphins which helps to create a sense of well-being and provides a total body workout.*

Spirituality

Spirituality has different connotations to individuals but many incorporate religion and prayers into their daily lives and find it very beneficial. [3]

* https://www.urmc.rochester.edu/encyclopedia/content.aspx?contenttypeid=85&contentid=p07338erapy
https://www.ncbi.nlm.nih.gov/pmc/articles/PMC4790847/

Summary

"Caring for your body, mind, and spirit is your greatest and grandest responsibility. It's about listening to the needs of your soul and then honoring them."

— Kristi Ling

It is empowering to know that you can take control of your health and well-being by learning about complementary therapies and different self-care practices. The integration of eastern medicine and western medicine is considered the best of both worlds. There are many benefits of modern medicine (aka Western medicine) which should not be ignored as many diseases and disorders have substantial research regarding evidence-based practices in diagnostics and therapeutics. The integration of the various self-care modalities and complementary therapies (Eastern medicine) may have a positive effect on your health outcomes. For example, when diagnosed with high blood pressure (hypertension) it is often treated with medication, however, lifestyle changes such as diet and exercise, stress management, decreasing salt, and smoking cessation are also recommended. Incorporating one or more of the self-care modalities can help to manage stress, lower blood pressure, and give you a feeling of well-being. The use of herbal teas has been shown to treat a variety of ailments so it is important to learn about them so you can choose which ones are best suited for your needs. Many of the self-care practices have been in existence for hundreds or even thousands of years but they have not been well researched, however, there is research to show many of the potential benefits. This is true with essential oils, too. You can use this book as a guide and then do your own research to learn more about the ones you are most interested in using. Although some of the healing modalities require a professionally trained healthcare practitioner such as hypnosis, ayurveda, and reiki therapy, many of them can be learned and incorporated into your health and wellness regimen. You may choose to do some, or all the self-care practices included in this book, but it is important to check with your healthcare provider before starting your self-care journey. I have used many practices in this book, and they have had a life changing effect on my body, mind, and spirit. However, this has been a journey, and I have spent many years learning about them and trying out different ones to see which ones work best for me. I hope you find this book helpful. I wish you much joy and wellness throughout your life.

Thank you for reading this book. I hope you found it beneficial. I would love to hear from you so please contact me on my website https://writerdebdolanhunt.com/contact/ Please share what you found helpful, your self-care practices or folk remedies that have been passed down from your family.

Notes

Herbal Teas

1. https://www.webmd.com/diet/health-benefits-blue berry-tea#1

https://www.livestrong.com/article/24647-blue berry-tea-benefits/

https://gtslivingfoods.com/faq/raw-kombucha/

https://www.verywellhealth.com/the-benefits-of-dan delion-root-89103

https://www.mayoclinic.org/healthy-lifestyle/con sumer-health/expert-answers/kombucha-tea/faq-20058126

https://www.forbes.com/sites/christinatroitino/2017/02/01/kombucha-101-demystifying-the-past-present-and-future-of-the-fermented-tea-drink/?sh=bdee6444ae24

https://www.healthline.com/nutrition/how-much-green-tea-per-day#TOC_TITLE_HDR_4n-tea

https://www.healthline.com/nutrition/rosehip-tea#

https://www.webmd.com/diet/licorice-root-tea-is-it-good-for-you#1

https://www.dilmahtea.com/herbal-infusion-tea/herbal-tea-benefits/rosehip.html

McKay DL, Blumberg JB. A review of the bioactivity and potential health benefits of peppermint tea (Mentha piperita L.)

Phytother Res. 2006 Aug;20(8):619-33. doi: 10.1002/ptr.1936. PMID: 16767798.

Notes

https://www.tasteofhome.com/article/peppermint-tea/

https://www.medicalnewstoday.com/articles/325242#tension-headaches

https://www.healthline.com/health/food-nutrition/benefits-ginger-tea#pain-relief

https://www.medicalnewstoday.com/articles/318120

https://www.medicalnewstoday.com/articles/318120#nutrition

https://www.verywellhealth.com/health-benefits-of-hibiscus-tea-89620

https://www.healthline.com/nutrition/echinacea#bottom-line

https://www.healthline.com/nutrition/echinacea#bottom-line

https://www.healthline.com/nutrition/licorice-root#side-effects

https://gardentherapy.ca/echinacea-root-and-flower-tincture/

https://wellnessmama.com/25999/echinacea-benefits-uses/

https://www.medicalnewstoday.com/articles/305576

https://www.hopkinsmedicine.org/health/wellness-and-prevention/ayurveda

https://www.healthline.com/nutrition/benefits-of-flaxseeds#TOC_TITLE_HDR_1

https://www.medicalnewstoday.com/articles/291334#_noHeaderPrefixedContent

https://simplelooseleaf.com/blog/black-tea/chai-tea-benefits/

https://www.medicalnewstoday.com/articles/291334#tips

Tinctures & Supplements

1. https://healthyeating.sfgate.com/benefits-turmeric-tincture-11310.html

   https://www.healthline.com/nutrition/reishi-mushroom-benefits

   https://www.medicalnewstoday.com/articles/323637#7-potential-health-benefits

   https://www.healthline.com/health/what-is-a-tincture

Healthy Super Foods

1. https://www.cnn.com/2017/04/18/health/apple-cider-vinegar-uses/index.html

   https://www.organicfacts.net/health-benefits/fruit/health-benefits-of-avocado.html

   https://www.organicfacts.net/health-benefits/fruit/health-benefits-of-lemon.html

   https://www.organicfacts.net/health-benefits/vegetable/cucumber.html

   https://www.healthline.com/nutrition/10-proven-benefits-of-kale

   https://www.livestrong.com/article/167554-side-effects-of-raw-honey/

   https://www.webmd.com/vitamins-supplements/ingredientmono-1468-quinoa.aspx?activeingredientid=1468&activeingredientname=quinoa

   https://www.organicfacts.net/health-benefits/vegetable/tomatoes.html

   https://www.healthline.com/nutrition/10-healthy-herbs-and-spices#modal-close

https://www.organicfacts.net/health-benefits/herbs-and-spices/health-benefits-of-cardamom.html

https://www.healthline.com/nutrition/10-proven-benefits-of-cinnamon

https://www.healthline.com/nutrition/side-effects-of-cinnamon

https://www.organicfacts.net/health-benefits/vegetable/cucumber.html

https://www.livestrong.com/article/527901-benefits-and-side-effects-of-cucumbers/

https://www.healthline.com/nutrition/11-proven-health-benefits-of-garlic

https://www.webmd.com/vitamins-supplements/ingredientmono-311-fennel.aspx?activeingredientid=311&activeingredientname=fennel

https://www.organicfacts.net/health-benefits/vegetable/cucumber.html

https://www.healthline.com/nutrition/10-proven-benefits-of-kale#section7

https://www.mybeeline.co/en/p/raw-honey-vs-regular-honey-difference

http://.com/2852/21-fantastic-benefits-of-cacao/

https://www.healthline.com/nutrition/8-benefits-of-cayenne-pepper#section1

https://www.healthline.com/nutrition/dragon-fruit-benefits#TOC_TITLE_HDR_8

https://www.webmd.com/vitamins-supplements/ingredientmono-961-GINGER.aspx

https://www.organicfacts.net/health-benefits/herbs-and-spices/health-benefits-of-parsley.html

https://www.organicfacts.net/health-benefits/herbs-and-spices/rosemary.html

https://www.organicfacts.net/health-benefits/herbs-and-spices/sage.html

https://www.webmd.com/vitamins-supplements/ingredientmono-662-turmeric.aspx?activeingredientid=662&activeingredientname=turmeric

https://www.webmd.com/vitamins-supplements/ingredientmono-961-GINGER.aspx

https://www.webmd.com/vitamins-supplements/ingredientmono-154-ROSEMARY.aspx?activeIngredientId=154&activeIngredientName=ROSEMARY

https://www.nccih.nih.gov/health/complementary-alternative-or-integrative-health-whats-in-a-name

https://www.webmd.com/vitamins/ai/ingredientmono-960/gree

Supplements & Vitamins

1. https://www.healthline.com/nutrition/8-health-benefits-of-probiotics#TOC_TITLE_HDR_8

Journaling and Cognitive-Behavioral Therapy

1. https://www.urmc.rochester.edu/encyclopedia/content.aspx?ContentID=4552&ContentTypeID=1

https://www.medicalnewstoday.com/articles/296579

https://healthypsych.com/psychology-tools-schedule-worry-time/

Complementary Therapy

1. https://www.1fur1.org/difference-animal-assisted-therapy-aat-activities-aaa-part-1-2/

Notes

2. https://www.healthline.com/health/anxiety/do-weighted-blankets-work#benefits
   https://www.pennmedicine.org/updates/blogs/health-and-wellness/2019/february/weighted-blankets
   https://www.mayoclinic.org/healthy-lifestyle/consumer-health/in-depth/pet-therapy/art-20046342
3. https://moonmagic.com/blogs/news/healing-stones

About the Author

Deborah Dolan Hunt, PhD, RN

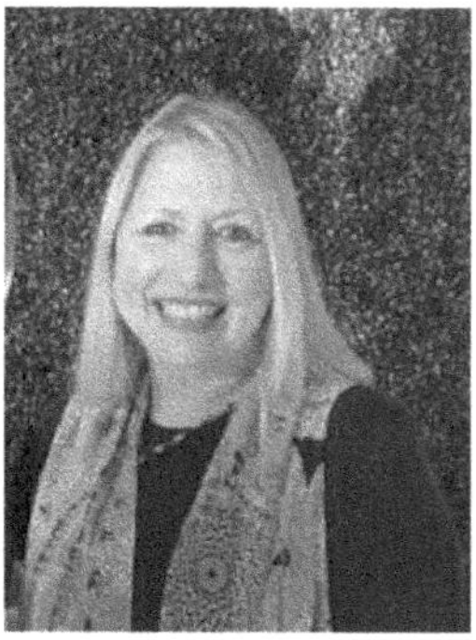

Deborah is a writer and nursing professor who lives in New York with her family. Deborah holds a PhD in nursing and has completed coursework related to many of the self-care modalities that are included in this book. Deborah is a health advocate and believes in an integrative approach to health and wellness. She refers to herself as an eclectic author as she writes in several genres. Her current book **Detective Natty and Doggy Dale Follow the Clues** was published by Clear Fork Press. Deborah loves meatballs and enjoys the beach, hiking, cooking, painting, gardening and hopes to own a farm one day. She loves sharing her books and hopes to inspire kids to love books just as much as she does.

"May you always have a book to read and a story to hold in your heart"

— D.D. Hunt

https://writerdebdolanhunt.com/

www.ingramcontent.com/pod-product-compliance
Lightning Source LLC
LaVergne TN
LVHW050936210926
848482LV00013B/629